FOLLOW-UP OF CANCER

A Handbook for Physicians

DAVID S. FISCHER, M.D.

Clinical Professor of Medicine, Yale University School of Medicine
Attending Physician, Yale New Haven Hospital
Emeritus Physician, Hospital of St. Raphael
New Haven, Connecticut

UNDER THE AUSPICES OF
American Cancer Society, Connecticut Division, Inc.
Connecticut State Department of Health Services
Connecticut State Medical Society
Yale Cancer Center

WITH 85 CONSULTANTS

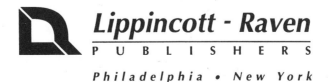

Lippincott - Raven
PUBLISHERS
Philadelphia • New York

Developmental Editor: Eileen Wolfberg
Production Editor: Virginia Barishek
Interior Designer: Berliner, Inc.
Cover Designer: Ilene Griff
Production: Berliner, Inc.
Printer/Binder: Courier Book Company/Kendallville
Cover Printer: Lehigh Press

Fourth Edition

Follow-up of cancer : a handbook for physicians / [edited by] David S.
    Fischer : under the auspices of American Cancer Society, Connecticut
    Division, Inc. . . . [et al.] : with 85 consultants. — 4th ed.
        p.   cm.
    Includes bibliographical references.
    ISBN 0-397-51533-2 (alk. paper)
    1. Cancer — Treatment — Handbooks. manuals, etc. 2. Cancer —
Relapse — Prevention — Handbooks, manuals, etc. 3. Cancer — Patients —
Long-term care — Handbooks, manuals, etc. I. Fischer, David S.
II. American Cancer Society. Connecticut Division.
    [DNLM : 1. Neoplasms — diagnosis — handbooks.   2. Follow-up Studies —
handbooks.   QZ 39 F668 1996]
RC270.8.F65   1996
616 .99' 406 — dc20
DNLM/DLC
for Library of Congress   95-31124
                                                                      CIP

⊗   This paper meets the requirements of ANSI/NISO Z39.48-1992 (permanence of paper).

        The material contained in this volume was submitted as previously unpublished mater-
ial, except in the instances in which credit has been given to the source from which some of the
illustrative material was derived.
        Great care has been taken to maintain the accuracy of the information contained in
the volume. However, neither Lippincott–Raven Publishers nor the editors can be held responsible for errors or for any consequences arising from the use of the information herein.
        The authors and publisher have exerted every effort to ensure that drug selection and
dosage set forth in this text are in accord with current recommendations and practice at the
time of publication. However, in view of ongoing research, changes in government regulations,
and the constant flow of information relating to drug therapy and drug reactions, the reader is
urged to check the package insert for each drug for any change in indications and dosage and
for added warnings and precautions. This is particularly important when the recommended
agent is a new or infrequently employed drug.
        Materials appearing in this book prepared by individuals as part of their official duties
as U.S. Government employees are not covered by the above mentioned copyright.

9   8   7   6   5   4   3   2   1

CONSULTANTS

DAN A. AVRADOPOULOS, M.D.
Fellow in Surgical Oncology
Roger Williams Medical Center
Providence, Rhode Island

NEIL H. BANDER, M.D.
Bernard & Josephine Chaus Chair
Director, Urologic Oncology
New York Hospital-Cornell Medical Center
New York, New York

G. PETER BEARDSLEY, PH.D., M.D.
Professor, Departments of Pediatrics &
    Pharmacology
Chief, Pediatric Hematology/Oncology
Yale University School of Medicine
New Haven, Connecticut

ROSS S. BERKOWITZ, M.D.
William H. Baker Professor Gynecology
Harvard Medical School
Co-Director, New England Trophoblastic
    Disease Center
Division of Gynecologic Oncology
Department of Obstetrics and Gynecology
Brigham and Women's Hospital
Boston, Massachusetts

PHILIP K. BONDY, M.D.
Professor Emeritus
Department of Medicine
Yale University School of Medicine
New Haven, Connecticut

GEORGE J. BOSL, M.D.
Head, Division of Solid Tumor Oncology
Memorial Sloan-Kettering Cancer Center
New York, New York

IRWIN M. BRAVERMAN, M.D.
Professor of Dermatology
Yale University School of Medicine
New Haven, Connecticut

ROBERT M. BYERS, M.D.
Alando J. Ballantyne Professor
Professor and Deputy Chairman
Department of Head & Neck Surgery
The University of Texas M.D. Anderson Cancer
    Center
Houston, Texas

PAUL CALABRESI, M.D.
Professor and Chairman Emeritus
Department of Medicine
Brown University School of Medicine
Providence, Rhode Island

GEORGE P. CANELLOS, M.D.
William Rosenberg Professor of Medicine
Harvard Medical School
Chief, Division of Medical Oncology
Dana-Farber Cancer Institute
Boston, Massachusetts

EPHRAIM S. CASPER, M.D.
Attending Physician, Gastrointestinal Oncology
    Service
Division of Solid Tumor Oncology, Department of
    Medicine
Memorial Sloan-Kettering Cancer Center
New York, New York

NICHOLAS J. CASSISI, M.D.
Professor and Chairman
Department of Otolaryngology
University of Florida College of Medicine
Gainesville, Florida

ROBERT P. CASTLEBERRY, JR., M.D.
Professor of Pediatrics
Director of Pediatric Hematology/Oncology
University of Alabama at Birmingham
Children's Hospital
Birmingham, Alabama

ABRAHAM CHACHOUA, M.D.
Research Assistant Professor of Medicine
New York University Medical Center
New York, New York

ALFRED M. COHEN, M.D.
Chief, Colorectal Service
Department of Surgery
Memorial Sloan-Kettering Cancer Center
Professor of Surgery
Cornell University Medical College
New York, New York

CARMEL J. COHEN, M.D.
Professor & Vice Chairman
Department of Obstetrics, Gynecology and
    Reproductive Sciences
Director, Division of Gynecologic Services
Mount Sinai School of Medicine
New York, New York

DENNIS COOPER, M.D.
Associate Professor of Medicine (Oncology)
Yale University School of Medicine
New Haven, Connecticut

WILLIAM T. CREASMAN, M.D.
Sims-Hester Professor and Chairman
Department of Obstetrics & Gynecology
Medical University of South Carolina
Charleston, South Carolina

GIULIO D'ANGIO, M.D.
Professor of Radiation Oncology
Pediatric Oncology and Radiology Emeritus
Department of Radiation Oncology
University of Pennsylvania School of Medicine
Philadelphia, Pennsylvania

VINCENT T. DEVITA, JR., M.D.
Director, Yale Comprehensive Cancer Center
Professor of Medicine (Oncology)
Yale University School of Medicine
New Haven, Connecticut

PHILLIP M. DEVLIN, M.D.
Resident in Radiation Oncology
Department of Radiation Oncology
University of Pennsylvania
Philadelphia, Pennsylvania

ÖZDAL DILLIOGLUGIL, M.D.
Urological Oncology Fellow
Scott Department of Urology
Baylor College of Medicine
Houston, Texas

SARAH S. DONALDSON, M.D.
Catherine and Howard Avery Professor of Radiation
    Oncology
Stanford University School of Medicine
Chief of Radiation Oncology Service
Lucille Salter Packard Children's Hospital at Stanford
Stanford, California

EDWIN C. DOUGLASS, M.D.
Director Clinical Oncology
Department of Pediatrics
Division of Hematology-Oncology
St. Christopher's Hospital for Children
Professor of Pediatrics
Temple University School of Medicine
Philadelphia, Pennsylvania

THOMAS P. DUFFY, M.D.
Professor of Medicine (Hematology)
Yale University School of Medicine
New Haven, Connecticut

LAWRENCE H. EINHORN, M.D.
Distinguished Professor of Medicine
Indiana University Medical Center
Indiana University Hospital
Indianapolis, Indiana

DAVID ESRIG, M.D.
Assistant Professor of Surgery (Urology)
Director, Urologic Oncology
Yale University School of Medicine
New Haven, Connecticut

WILLIAM R. FAIR, M.D.
Chief, Urologic Surgery, Florence and Theodore
    Baumritter/Enid Ancell Chair of Urologic
    Oncology
Memorial Sloan-Kettering Cancer Center
New York, New York

WILLARD E. FEE, JR., M.D.
Professor and Chairman
Division of Otolaryngology-Head and Neck Surgery
Stanford University Medical Center
Stanford, California

GARY E. FRIEDLAENDER, M.D.
Professor and Chairman
Department of Orthopaedics and Rehabilitation
Yale University School of Medicine
New Haven, Connecticut

ALVIN E. FRIEDMAN-KIEN, M.D.
Professor of Dermatology and Microbiology
New York University Medical Center
New York, New York

DAVID M. GERSHENSON, M.D.
Professor and Deputy Chairman
Department of Gynecologic Oncology
University of Texas M.D. Anderson Cancer Center
Houston, Texas

JEFFREY M. GOLDBERG, M.D.
Fellow, Department of Gynecologic Oncology
Roswell Park Cancer Institute
Assistant Clinical Instructor of Obstetrics and
    Gynecology
State University of New York at Buffalo
School of Medicine and Biomedical Sciences
Buffalo, New York

DONALD P. GOLDSTEIN, M.D.
Assistant Clinical Professor of Obstetrics
Gynecology and Reproductive Biology
Harvard Medical School
Director, New England Trophoblastic Disease Center
Division of Gynecologic Oncology
Department of Obstetrics and Gynecology
Brigham and Women's Hospital
Boston, Massachusetts

JEROME C. GOLDSTEIN, M.D.
Executive Vice President
American Academy of Otolaryngology-Head and
    Neck Surgery
Adjunct Professor of Otolaryngology
Johns Hopkins University and Georgetown University
Washington, D.C.

HARVEY M. GOLOMB, M.D.
Professor, Department of Medicine
Director, Section of Hematology/Oncology
University of Chicago
Pritzker School of Medicine
Chicago, Illinois

STEVEN M. GRUNBERG, M.D.
Professor of Medicine
Vermont Cancer Center
University of Vermont
Burlington, Vermont

HOWARD D. HOMESLEY, M.D.
Professor and Head
Section on Gynecologic Oncology
The Bowman Gray School of Medicine of Wake
    Forest University
Winston-Salem, North Carolina

WILLIAM J. HOSKINS, M.D.
Chief, Gynecology Service
Memorial Sloan-Kettering Cancer Center
New York, New York

ROGER I. JENKINS, M.D.
Associate Professor of Surgery
Harvard Medical School
Chief, Division of Hepatobiliary Surgery and Liver
    Transplantation
Deaconess Hospital
Boston, Massachusetts

DAVID P. KELSEN, M.D.
Chief, Gastrointestinal Oncology Service
Department of Medicine
Memorial Sloan-Kettering Cancer Center
New York, New York

DIANE M. KOMP, M.D.
Professor of Pediatrics (Hematology/Oncology)
Yale University School of Medicine
New Haven, Connecticut

LARRY K. KVOLS, M.D.
Director, Clinical Research
Mallinckrodt Medical Inc.
Professor of Clinical Medicine
Washington University School of Medicine
St. Louis, Missouri

ROBERT A. KYLE, M.D.
Professor of Medicine and Laboratory Medicine
Mayo Medical School
Rochester, Minnesota

ALEXANDRA M. LEVINE, M.D.
Professor of Medicine
Chief, Division of Hematology
USC Norris Cancer Hospital
University of Southern California School of Medicine
Los Angeles, California

PETER E. LIGGETT, M.D.
Professor of Ophthalmology
Yale University School of Medicine
New Haven, Connecticut

MICHAEL P. LINK, M.D.
Professor of Pediatrics
Division of Hematology/Oncology
Stanford University School of Medicine
Lucille Salter Packard Children's Hospital
Stanford, California

BERNARD LYTTON, M.D.
Donald Guthrie Professor of Surgery (Urology)
Yale University School of Medicine
New Haven, Connecticut

IAN T. MAGRATH, M.D.
Head, Lymphoma Biology Section
Pediatric Branch
National Cancer Institute
Bethesda, Maryland

HENRY J. MANKIN, M.D.
Chief, Orthopaedic Service
Massachusetts General Hospital
Edith M. Ashley Professor of Orthopaedic Surgery
Harvard Medical School
Boston, Massachusetts

JOHN C. MARSH, M.D.
Professor of Medicine (Oncology)
Lecturer in Pharmacology
Yale University School of Medicine
New Haven, Connecticut

WILLIAM M. MCCONAHEY, M.D.
Emeritus Professor of Medicine
Mayo Medical School
Rochester, Minnesota

CHARLES J. MCDONALD, M.D.
Professor and Director
Division of Dermatology
Brown University School of Medicine
Providence, Rhode Island

JAMES S. MISER, M.D.
Clinical Director, Hematology/Oncology
Children's Hospital and Medical Center
John R. Hartmann Associate Professor of Pediatric
    Hematology/Oncology
University of Washington School of Medicine
Seattle, Washington

IRVIN M. MODLIN, M.D., PH.D.
Professor of Surgery (Gastroenterology)
Director, GI Surgical Pathology Research Group
Yale University School of Medicine
New Haven, Connecticut

A. RAHIM MOOSSA, M.D.
Professor and Chairman
Department of Surgery
University of California School of Medicine at
    San Diego
Surgeon-in-Chief
University of California San Diego Medical Center
San Diego, California

MONICA MORROW, M.D.
Director, Lynn Sage Comprehensive Breast Center
Associate Professor of Surgery
Northwestern University School of Medicine
Chicago, Illinois

CHARLES M. NORRIS, JR., M.D.
Assistant Professor, Department of Otology and
    Laryngology
Harvard Medical School
Chief, Division of Otolaryngology-Head and Neck
    Surgery
New England Deaconess Hospital
Surgical Director, Head and Neck Oncology Program
Dana-Farber Cancer Institute
Boston, Massachusetts

ROGER J. PACKER, M.D.
Chairman, Department of Neurology
Children's National Medical Center
Professor of Neurology and Pediatrics
George Washington University School of Medicine
Washington, D.C.

HARVEY I. PASS, M.D.
Head, Thoracic Oncology Section
Senior Investigator, Surgery Branch
National Cancer Institute
Bethesda, Maryland

M. STEVEN PIVER, M.D.
Chief, Department Gynecologic Oncology
Roswell Park Cancer Institute
Professor of Gynecology
State University of New York at Buffalo School of
    Medicine and Biomedical Sciences
Buffalo, New York

DAVID G. POPLACK, M.D.
Elise C. Young Professor of Pediatric Oncology
Baylor College of Medicine
Director, Texas Children's Cancer Center
Texas Children's Hospital
Houston, Texas

JEROME B. POSNER, M.D.
George C. Cotzias Chair in Neuro-Oncology
Chairman, Department of Neurology
Memorial Sloan-Kettering Cancer Center
New York, New York

KANTI ROOP RAI, M.D.
Professor of Medicine
Albert Einstein College of Medicine
Chief, Division of Hematology/Oncology
Long Island Jewish Medical Center
New Hyde Park, New York

R. BEVERLY RANEY, JR., M.D.
Professor of Pediatrics, Deputy Head
Department of Pediatrics
University of Texas
M.D. Anderson Cancer Center
Houston, Texas

THANJAVUR S. RAVIKUMAR, M.D.
Professor of Surgery and Molecular Genetics
Robert Wood Johnson Medical School
Associate Director and Chief of Surgical Oncology
The Cancer Institute of New Jersey
New Brunswick, New Jersey

GERALD ROSEN, M.D.
Medical Director
The Cedars-Sinai Comprehensive Cancer Center
Los Angeles, California

JERRY C. ROSENBERG, M.D.
Professor of Surgery
Wayne State University
Chief of Surgery
Hutzel Hospital
Detroit, Michigan

STEVEN A. ROSENBERG, M.D.
Chief of Surgery
National Cancer Institute
Professor of Surgery
Uniformed Services University of the Health Sciences
Bethesda, Maryland

BIJAN SAFAI, M.D.
Professor and Chairman
Department of Dermatology
New York Medical College
Valhalla, New York

CLARENCE T. SASAKI, M.D.
Ohse Professor of Surgery
Chief, Section of Otolaryngology
Yale University School of Medicine
New Haven, Connecticut

PETER T. SCARDINO, M.D.
Russel and May Hugh Scott Professor and Chairman
Scott Department of Urology
Baylor College of Medicine
Houston, Texas

JOSEPH D. SCHMIDT, M.D.
Professor and Head
Division of Urology
University of California Medical Center at San Diego
San Diego, California

PETER E. SCHWARTZ, M.D.
Professor of Gynecologic Oncology
Vice-chairman and Director, Gynecologic Oncology
Yale University School of Medicine
New Haven, Connecticut

JONATHAN E. SEARS, M.D.
Resident, Department of Ophthalmology
Yale University School of Medicine
New Haven, Connecticut

ROY B. SESSIONS, M.D.
Professor and Chairman
Georgetown University Medical School
Chief of Otolaryngology-Head and Neck Surgery
Member, Vincent Lombardi Cancer Center
Georgetown University Medical Center
Washington, D.C.

AZIZA T. SHAD, M.D.
Assistant Professor of Pediatrics
Uniformed Services University of the Health Sciences
Pediatric Branch
National Cancer Institute
Bethesda, Maryland

WILLIAM F. SINDELAR, M.D.
Senior Investigator, Surgery Branch
National Cancer Institute
Bethesda, Maryland

JEFFREY D. SPIRO, M.D.
Associate Professor of Surgery
Division of Otolaryngology-Head and Neck Surgery
School of Medicine of the University of Connecticut
    Health Center
Farmington, Connecticut

GREGORY P. SUTTON, M.D.
Professor and Chief
Department of Obstetrics and Gynecology
Indiana University Medical Center
Indiana University Hospital
Indianapolis, Indiana

JOHN E. ULTMANN, M.D.
Professor, Department of Medicine
Director Emeritus
University of Chicago Cancer Research Center
University of Chicago School of Medicine
Chicago, Illinois

HAROLD J. WANEBO, M.D.
Professor of Surgery, Director of Surgical Oncology
Brown University School of Medicine
Chief of Surgery
Roger Williams Medical Center
Providence, Rhode Island

HOWARD J. WEINSTEIN, M.D.
Associate Professor of Pediatrics
Harvard Medical School
Director of Pediatric Bone Marrow Transplantation
Division of Pediatric Hematology-Oncology
Children's Hospital and the Dana-Farber Cancer
    Institute
Boston, Massachusetts

BARRY L. WENIG, M.D.
Associate Professor
Department of Otolaryngology-Head and Neck
    Surgery
Director, Division of Head and Neck Surgery
University of Illinois College of Medicine
Chicago, Illinois

PETER H. WIERNICK, M.D.
Professor of Medicine
Albert Einstein Cancer Center
Montefiore Medical Center
Bronx, New York

PREFACE

Although it is only 5 years since our third edition presented suggestions for follow-up of 30 cancer sites, some of these recommendations are outdated, and since we had exhausted our supply of the 20,000 copies printed, it seemed time for a new edition. Dr. Vincent T. DeVita, Jr., director of the Yale Cancer Center, suggested that the book be expanded to include additional cancer sites and contributions from consultants nationwide. Accordingly, I selected 76 cancer sites from the on-line Physician's Data Query (PDQ) and wrote a draft information page based on the Bibliography included in this book. I then sent it along with a suggested follow-up from our third edition (with some suggested modifications when appropriate) to national and international expert consultants and asked for their comments and modifications with special attention to cost-effectiveness and best medical care.

The 85 consultants are listed with the cancer site on which they commented. In a few cases (childhood brain tumors, Wilms' tumor, Kaposi's sarcoma, gestational trophoblastic tumors, chronic lymphocytic leukemia, testicular cancer, and extragonadal and gonadal tumors), the consultants largely rewrote the draft—at least the follow-up portion—and the author used their formulation. Almost all the material was reviewed by one or two of the editorial consultants for accuracy and appropriateness, but complete agreement is not possible as clearly we are dealing with the art of medicine as well as its science, and there are bound to be differences of opinion and style among equally experienced and knowledgeable physicians. However, all errors of omission or commission are my responsibility alone.

Listings of new cancer cases and estimated cancer deaths were taken from the American Cancer Society figures for 1994 when available. Since the manuscript was submitted, the 1995 estimates became available. They estimate 44,000 new cancer cases, with some increases and decreases for specific cancer sites. Significant changes were noted for lip, colon, rectum, prostate, and lung cancers and non-Hodgkin's lymphoma. Accordingly, the 1995 estimates are listed for these cancers. The 5-year relative survival rates by stage (localized, regional, distant) have been taken from the *SEER Twentieth Anniversary 1973–1993 Cancer Statistics Review* when available, which has the advantage of continuity of definition over 20 years and a very large database. Where these data were unavailable, the staging of the American Joint Committee on Cancer was used, with the advantage of greater precision of staging, but the disadvantage that some of the stage definitions have changed with each revision—1977, 1982, and 1988—and the latest (fourth) edition is 1992, which we used. In the very few cases in which neither was widely used, we used the system that was most widely selected in the literature.

How often should cancer patients be recalled for examination? What should be done at each visit? It is often difficult to remember each procedure or examination that might be done and then to decide which is important and which unnecessary, especially in tumors that one does not see frequently. What lifestyle modifications are indicated? What implications does the patient's malignancy have for genetic relatives and for further screening for other malignancies? What are the risk factors? We try to answer these questions within the limits of brief discussions.

The recommendations in this book are just that—suggestions to remind and assist the physician in follow-up, but in no way should they limit or completely direct the physician. They are *not* standards of minimum or optimum care. Each patient deserves a personalized follow-up. Patients with some neoplasms will need to see the appropriate specialist periodically in addition to the primary physician.

The included recommendations are reasonable, but they are the somewhat arbitrary preferences of one group of physicians and will have to be modified in consideration of stage and histologic type and changing information. Suggestions and corrections may be addressed via e-mail to dsfischer@aol.com or by fax to (203)882-8414 or by hard copy to Oncology Division, Medical Editorial Dept., Lippincott-Raven Publishers, 227 West Washington Square, Philadelphia PA 19106-3780. Patients with known residual cancer should be under the care of an oncologist. Family members at increased risk should be made aware of the situation as it impacts on them. In general, the matter of therapy is only addressed in passing, but the Bibliography heavily emphasizes it. Hopefully, better follow-up will lead to a better quality of life and longer survival for our patients.

David S. Fischer, M.D.

ACKNOWLEDGMENTS

I could not have completed the fourth edition of this book without the assistance of many people.

Dr. Vincent T. DeVita, Jr., director of the Yale Cancer Center (YCC), suggested the expansion of this edition and the enlistment of consultants from all over the United States.

Marion Morra, director of the Cancer Information Service (CIS) at YCC, Linda Mowad, manager of CIS; and Ann Bradley at CIS obtained bibliographical material for me, as did Susan Richter and David Woodmansie of the Connecticut division of the American Cancer Society. Majlen Helenius of the Yale Medical Library helped with accessing Medline, PDQ, and other on-line computer services. Louise E. Fischer set up my computer and coached me in its use. Dr. Jack Van Hoff, associate professor of pediatrics at Yale, made some pediatric oncology protocols available to me.

The 85 consultants who reviewed and corrected the drafts that I sent them and gave of their valuable time, in some cases rewriting the material, give this book the credibility to serve colleagues as a first-step reference source for recommendations on the follow-up of their cancer patients.

The editorial consultants, in addition to serving as consultants on one cancer site, also helped in the selection of other consultants in their fields and then reviewed the final material in their respective areas of expertise. In childhood diseases, Drs. Diane M. Komp and G. Peter Beardsley; in otolaryngology, Dr. Clarence T. Sasaki; in gynecology, Dr. Peter E. Schwartz; in orthopedics, Dr. Gary E. Friedlaender; in hematology, Dr. Thomas P. Duffy; in urology, Dr. Bernard Lytton; in gastroenterology, Dr. John C. Marsh. In addition, Dr. Marsh was kind enough to read all the didactic chapters and discuss some of the controversial material in them.

J. Stuart Freeman, Jr., senior editor, and Eileen Wolfberg, developmental editor, in the oncology program at Lippincott–Raven Publishers, were helpful, cooperative, and encouraging. It was a pleasure to work with them. Nancy Berliner of Berliner, Inc. improved the design and gave helpful suggestions.

Finally, I wish to acknowledge my patients, who taught me about courage and compassion as they struggled with this terrible disease; and my students, who asked the difficult questions that reinforced the concept that medical education is a lifelong endeavor. As we go forward with basic and clinical research, more of those questions will have better answers.

INTRODUCTION

"The goal of cancer therapy is cure, not 5-year survival. By cure, we now mean that the person afflicted will have an actuarial survival equal to that of an age-matched cohort who is free of cancer. Even to begin to approach this goal we need early diagnosis, definitive therapy, and a system of follow-up to detect recurrences while they are still curable or at least treatable." That is what I wrote for the introduction to the second edition of this manual published in 1983. The goal is as clear and important now as it was then. The definition of *cure* is a little more ambiguous. Can we apply the term *cured* to the patient with cancer who outlives the actuarial survival of the age-matched cohort but later dies of cancer; or to the cancer patient who is asymptomatic and apparently disease-free at nine annual competent examinations who then dies of a myocardial infarction and is found to have gross residual or metastatic cancer at autopsy? We have a semantic problem defining *cure*, but it is a happy problem of medical progress.

It is just over half a century since mechlorethamine (nitrogen mustard), which had been developed as a wartime poison gas, was first used at Yale–New Haven Hospital for the treatment of a lymphoma and an inoperable lung cancer. In 1948, methotrexate was first used at Boston Children's Hospital for acute leukemia, and in 1957, 5-fluorouracil was introduced at the University of Wisconsin for treatment of solid tumors. In the early 1960s, combination chemotherapy was reported for testicular cancer at Memorial Hospital in New York, for breast cancer at Mt. Sinai Hospital in New York, and for Hodgkin's disease at the National Cancer Institute at Bethesda. The reality of prolonging survival and even of producing cures was advanced with the validation of the value of adjuvant chemotherapy for breast cancer. The responses of neoplastic diseases to chemotherapy are listed in Table 1 and will get better as the role of high-dose chemotherapy with stem cell (and bone marrow) support and cytokines is clarified with more prospective randomized trials. Compared to a half century ago, when our major tools for cancer therapy were surgery and radiation therapy, our progress has been incredible. The improvements in surgical instrumentation and technique, combined with advances in endoscopy and diagnostic imaging and megavoltage radiation, promise even better results.

In spite of these advantages, many people disparage therapy that produces anything less than a cure and suggest that it is not worthwhile or even cost-effective. Without going into a philosophical discussion of what pain and suffering are worth, or what a human life is worth, suffice it to say that most people agree that prolongation of life of reasonably good quality is a societal benefit and a laudable goal. Hence, it is useful to review the course of a patient treated for cure when possible, or for prolongation and palliation when cure is not possible (Figure 1).

Unfortunately, at the present time the majority of the common malignancies and many of the less common ones are incurable at the time of diagnosis with the currently available armamentarium (see chapter on tumor markers for earlier diagnosis of recurrent disease, and the chapter on metastasis). Hence, our goals must be to provide therapy that will prolong survival with a high quality of life during the time of increased survival. Throughout this time, and when therapy ultimately fails, another goal must be the compassionate care of these patients and their families. What Dr. Francis Weld Peabody wrote in 1927, just before his own death from gastric cancer at age 45, is true today:

> The good physician knows his patient through and through, and his knowledge is bought dearly. Time, sympathy, and understanding must be lavishly dispensed, but the reward is to be found in that personal bond which forms the greatest satisfaction of the practice of medicine. One of the essential qualities of the clinician is interest in humanity, for the secret of the care of the patient is in caring for the patient. (JAMA 1927;88:877)

Physicians have spent much time and effort in sharpening their diagnostic and therapeutic skills. Somehow, though, it came to be regarded as crass and commercial for physicians to recall these cancer patients for follow-up, although dentists do it routinely.

On April 5, 1973, the Council of the Connecticut State Medical Society (CSMS) resolved that "it is both proper and advisable for the attending physician to call patients back for appropriate follow-

TABLE I. NEOPLASTIC DISEASES AND THEIR RESPONSE TO CHEMOTHERAPY

Type of cancer	% Therapeutic Response (PR + CR)	Survival of Responders
Prolonged survival or cure		
Gestational trophoblastic tumors	70–95	60% cured with high tumor burden
		90% cured with moderate tumor burden
Burkitt's tumor	>50–60	50% cured
Seminoma	95	90% cured
Nonseminomatous testicular	90	90% cured
Wilms' tumor	60–80	65% cured with adjuvant CT
Osteogenic sarcoma	60–80	65% cured with adjuvant CT
Neuroblastoma	50–80	>20% cured
Acute lymphocytic leukemia (adults)	50–60	30% cured
Acute lymphoblastic leukemia (children)	90	70% cured
Non-Hodgkin's lymphoma (children)	90	60% cured
Non-Hodgkin's (DLC) lymphoma (adults)	75	50% cured
Rhabdomyosarcoma	90	70% cured with adjuvant CT
Hodgkin's disease	90	80% cured
Acute myelogenous leukemia	50–80	15% cured
Palliation and prolongation of survival		
Prostate cancer	70	Increased
Breast cancer	60	Increased with adjuvant CT
Chronic lymphocytic leukemia	50	Slightly increased
Non-Hodgkin's indolent lymphoma (adults)	60	Increased
Multiple myeloma	60	Slightly increased
Small-cell carcinoma of the lung	60	2–5% cured
Chronic myelocytic leukemia	90	Increased
Palliation with uncertain prolongation of life		
Ovarian cancer	30–50	Probably increased
Endometrial cancer	25	Probably increased
Soft tissue sarcoma	30–50	Probably increased with adjuvant CT
Gastric cancer	30	Probably increased
Colorectal cancer	30–40	Increased with adjuvant CT
Anal cancer (CT + RT)	70	Probably increased
Bladder cancer	30–40	Probably increased
Uncertain palliation		
Pancreatic cancer	10–15	Brief
Liver cancer	10–15	Brief
Cervical cancer	20	Brief
Melanoma (cutaneous)	20	Brief
Adrenal cortical cancer	20	Brief
Kidney cancer	10–20	Brief

Abbreviations: CT, chemotherapy; RT, radiation therapy; PR, partial response; CR, complete response; DLC, diffuse large cell.

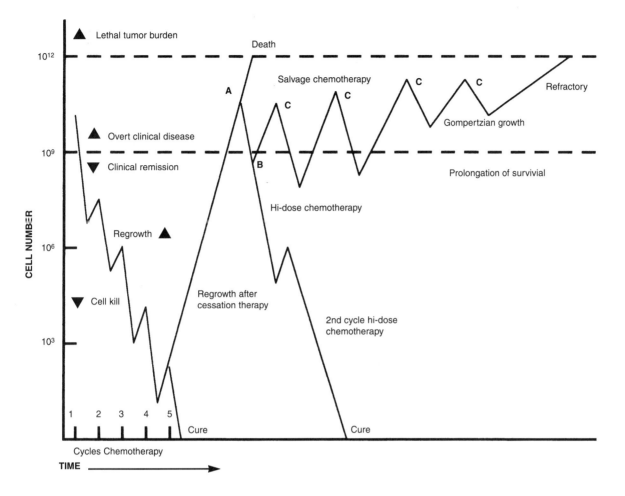

FIGURE 1. The relationship between tumor burden and chemotherapy and the potential for increased survival or cure is illustrated. If a patient with a clinically overt neoplasm (non-Hodgkin's disease in this hypothetical example) is treated for four cycles of chemotherapy, the tumor burden decreases by a roughly standard amount with each treatment and regrows a little between each treatment, but the patient remains in clinical remission with no evidence of disease. If therapy ceases at this point in time, before the patient is cured, the tumor will regrow, and in the continued absence of therapy, will lead to death as it exceeds the lethal tumor burden. If the patient is treated for a fifth cycle, when the tumor burden is very low and the immune system is still not significantly impaired, cure is possible. If the patient had treatment interrupted until disease was clinically overt (A), and was retreated with the same or a similar regimen, then the tumor might shrink (B) but regrow. With salvage chemotherapy, cycles of shrinkage and growth would continue (C) until the tumor burden became large and began to grow more slowly (Gompertzian growth), but with less response to therapy until it became refractory and the patient died. If at the point of recurrent overt clinical disease (A) the patient were treated with high-dose (ablative) therapy with stem cell (bone marrow) support, a much larger cell death would occur and cure might occur directly, or more likely with a second high-dose course of chemotherapy. In either case, the follow-up to detect the recurrence would have led to either cure or prolongation of survival. (Modified and expanded from Cooper MR, Cooper MR, in Holleb IA, Fink DJ, Murphy GP, eds, Textbook of Clinical Oncology. Atlanta: American Cancer Society, 1991, 53.)

up examination … this is not an unethical practice but, in fact, quite the contrary." CSMS urged that physicians, hospitals, and the public be so informed, and that the cooperation of the Connecticut division of the American Cancer Society (ACS) be enlisted in sponsoring this practice and in pointing out to the public "its value to patients" in the treatment of malignant disease.

As a result of this impetus, an effort was begun in 1973 by the CSMS and ACS with the cooperation of the Connecticut State Department of Health, which maintains the Connecticut Tumor Registry, the oldest population-based cancer registry in the world (collecting data since 1935). Using the resources of the three groups, it was decided to publish a manual for physicians following cancer patients. An editorial committee sought the advice and expertise of 57 physicians and specialists and came up with recommendations (not standards) to assist in the cancer follow-up of 11 major solid tumor sites (Bradley ET, Barrett HS, eds, Follow-up of Cancer: A Handbook for Physicians. New Haven, CT: ACS, 1974).

In 1976, the Commission on Cancer of the American College of Surgeons published *The Patient with Cancer: guidelines for follow-up*, based on the Connecticut manual, but expanded to cover 21 sites. In 1983, I had the privilege of editing the second edition of *Follow-up of Cancer*, based on an update of the material of a chapter I wrote for *Cancer Therapy* (Fischer DS, Marsh JC, Cancer Therapy. Boston: G. K. Hall, 1982). The Yale Cancer Center joined the three other sponsors of the manual for its second and subsequent editions. In 1989, I edited the third edition with additional consultants and expanded to cover 30 sites. After the manuscript was completed, Linda Mowad of the Cancer Information Service at Yale called my attention to *Follow-up of the Cancer Patient* (by WA Robinson and G Steele, Jr. New York: Thieme-Stratton, 1982). This book is excellent but somewhat outdated.

There are two phases to follow-up. Continued assessment of the malignant disease is, of course, vital and somewhat scientific, but follow-up of the patient as a person is equally important. Whether or not the physician who administered the definitive treatment continues to see the patient periodically, the family physician is urged to maintain a strong supportive relationship with the patient and the family. Emotional support is essential. The physician can often aid in job rehabilitation and social reintegration in the community, and provide guidance to other resources.

Disaster may result from the patient being lost to follow-up. To avoid such tragedy, and to help make important statistical analyses valid for public health information, careful cooperation is necessary between the family physician and the physician (and hospital) responsible for definitive therapy, lest each assume the other to be following the patient and neither seeing the patient. They should be specific with each other and with the patient. In fact, the patient must be an active partner in follow-up, should be impressed with the importance of keeping recall appointments, and should be urged to report early and promptly any significant signs and symptoms.

The risk of a second primary tumor in the same or a different organ is higher in individuals who have already had one cancer. Attention during follow-up is therefore also directed toward early detection of new disease, recognition of recurrent disease, amelioration of posttherapy toxicity (see the chapter on late and delayed toxicity), and guidance in lifestyle modifications that may reduce the risk of new malignancies (see the chapters on prevention and on guidelines for the cancer-related checkup, although these issues are controversial).

In addition to the recommendations for follow-up of each specific site, it is good practice to also check the Recommendations for the Early Detection of Cancer in the chart of the ACS on page 161. Although some of the site recommendations in this book include the ACS recommendations, in general we did not repeat them for every site, assuming that they are generally applicable to all sites and do not require repetition. We also assume that all histories will include questions about tobacco usage, the most common cause of preventable death in the United States and probably in the world.

We hope that this book will aid physicians to help cancer patients to be cured or to increase their quality of life. The future of cancer therapy looks promising, but a cancer prevented is much better than a cancer cured.

David S. Fischer, M.D.

CONTENTS

FOLLOW-UP OF CANCER

OF

CANCER

A Handbook for Physicians

CENTRAL NERVOUS SYSTEM CANCER

CONSULTANT: *Jerome B. Posner, M.D.—Neurologist*

Primary CNS tumors (those that arise in the CNS and are not metastatic to it) make up 1% of all cancers in the United States and cause 2.5% of cancer deaths. Mortality rates and survival rates vary with tumor type. Staging is useful only in those tumors that commonly seed the neuraxis, eg, medulloblastoma. For example, the 5-year survival of patients with glioblastoma is less than 5%, whereas the 5-year survival for those with medulloblastoma is 60%. Local spread is common in the more malignant tumors but extracranial metastases are rare in all CNS tumors.

INCIDENCE AND SURVIVAL

	Total	Male	Female
Incidence rate per 100,000/yr	14.1	14.0	14.2
New cancer cases (ACS est 1994)	17,500	9600	7900
Cancer deaths (ACS est 1994)	12,600	6800	5800

Trends

The incidence has increased over the past two decades, particularly among the elderly. The increased incidence is particularly prominent in primary CNS lymphoma, less so in gliomas in the elderly. Because CNS tumors in elderly patients have a poor prognosis, mortality has increased as well.

Major risk factors

Ionizing radiation, hereditary syndromes, immunosuppression (lymphoma). No environmental risk factors have unequivocally been identified as causal in CNS tumors.

Pathology (major types)

Astrocytomas, anaplastic astrocytomas, glioblastoma multiforme, ependymomas, oligodendrogliomas, mixed glial tumors, medulloblastomas, pineal parenchymal tumors, germ cell tumors, lymphomas, meningiomas, and pituitary adenomas.

Metastatic sites (major)

CNS tumors rarely metastasize outside the nervous system. Neuraxis spread via CSF pathways occurs with medulloblastoma, lymphoma, germ cell and pineal tumors, and ependymomas.

Therapy

Surgery, radiation, and chemotherapy.

Recommendations to family

Obtain genetic counseling for hereditary tumors.

FOLLOW-UP OF THE PATIENT WITH CENTRAL NERVOUS SYSTEM CANCER

	1st Year (Months)				2nd–5th Year (Months)		Thereafter (Months)
	3	6	9	12	6	12	12
History							
Complete				×	×		×
Headache	×	×	×		×		
Seizures	×	×	×		×		
Mental changes	×	×	×		×		
Motor deficit	×	×	×		×		
Speech changes	×	×	×		×		
Balance problems							
Physical							
Complete				×	×		×
Cranial nerves	×	×	×		×		
Motor exam	×	×	×		×		
Sensory exam	×	×	×		×		
Gait	×	×	×		×		
Fundi	×	×	×		×		
Tests							
Chest x-ray	As indicated						
CBC (no chemotherapy)	As indicated						
MRI	×	×	×	×	×		×

Comments: With the development and wider availability of magnetic resonance imaging (MRI), earlier diagnosis of brain tumors is now possible. This has resulted in better surgical results and longer survivals, especially in low-grade tumors such as astrocytomas, meningiomas, ependymomas, and oligodendrogliomas. Treatment of high-grade tumors like glioblastoma multiforme is still discouraging, but increased survival duration and quality have accrued from multimodal therapy with surgery, radiation, chemotherapy, and corticosteroids. Careful follow-up is especially important in those who have had a long disease-free interval because relapse can sometimes be treated effectively with another therapeutic intervention.

At one time, all patients with brain tumors were maintained on anticonvulsants prophylactically. Now, some recommend anticonvulsants, primarily in patients who have had a seizure, and only in special circumstances as prophylaxis.

Skull x-rays, EEG, and CT scans are rarely indicated in follow-up of brain tumors.

RETINOBLASTOMA (RB)

CONSULTANTS: Peter E. Liggett, M.D.—Ophthalmic Surgeon
Jonathan E. Sears, M.D.—Ophthalmic Surgeon

Retinoblastoma is the most common intraocular malignancy in childhood, occurring in from 1 in 14,000 to 1 in 20,000 live births, with 250–300 new cases reported per year in the United States. Average age at diagnosis is 15 months for bilateral disease and 24 months for unilateral disease.

Major risk factors

Ninety percent are diagnosed before the age of 3 years. The tumor has no racial or gender predilection. It occurs bilaterally in 35% of affected patients. Sixty percent of patients present with leukocoria; 22% present with strabismus. A few percent of patients initially seek an ophthalmologist for orbital inflammation and proptosis, or the sequelae from neovascularization of the iris that can cause a spontaneous hyphema or a red painful eye from secondary glaucoma.

Pathology

A neuroblastic cancer that histologically demonstrates Flexner-Wintersteiner rosettes containing small, round cells with hyperchromatic nuclei and scant cytoplasm that attempt to form photoreceptor aggregates around blood vessels. Calcification and necrosis can be seen. The tumor can be endophytic, growing into the vitreous; or exophytic, growing in the subretinal space, causing retinal detachment and creating a white pupillary reflex.

Metastatic sites (major)

Extraocular extension of the tumor can occur by direct extension through the sclera, by hematogenous spread, or by passage of tumor cells into the optic nerve where they gain access to the subarachnoid space. Both hematogenous and lymphatic metastases occur to the marrow of the skull and distant bones and to lymph nodes and viscera. At autopsy, 23% have spinal cord metastases. A variant involves the pineal gland in some patients with bilateral eye disease, resulting in trilateral retinoblastoma.

Associated malignancies

Patients are at risk for secondary tumors such as osteosarcoma, various soft tissue sarcomas, malignant melanoma, leukemia and lymphoma, and various brain tumors. Two-thirds of the osteosarcomas occur within the treated radiation field.

Therapy

Treatment includes cobalt plaque irradiation, external beam irradiation, and chemotherapy.

Recommendations to family

Seek genetic counseling. Forty percent of new patients with RB have heritable disease and require genetic counseling. Six percent of patients have an autosomal dominant pattern with close to 90% penetrance. The remaining 94% occur without family history; 25% are heritable and 75% are a somatic mutation. Either the absence of or a defect in chromosome 13 at q14 predisposes to oncogenesis. An abnormal genotype can be found in germ cells (heritable disease) or only in tumor cells (somatic). A single normal copy of the suppressor gene rescues the abnormal genotype. The importance of screening the leukocytes of affected children is to determine whether the abnormality is carried by all somatic cells, thereby proving that it is a germ line mutation with consequences for the remainder of the family, and of prognostic importance for the future evolution of the patient's disease.

FOLLOW-UP OF THE PATIENT WITH RETINOBLASTOMA

	1st Year (Months)		2nd–7th Year (Months)		Thereafter (Months)
	6	12	6	12	12
PRIMARY PEDIATRICIAN					
History					
Complete	X	X	X	X	X
Vision	X	X	X	X	X
Development	X	X	X	X	X
Bone pain	X	X	X	X	X
GI discomfort	X	X	X	X	X
Physical					
Complete	X	X	X	X	X
Neurological exam	X	X	X	X	X
Abdomen	X	X	X	X	X
Lymph nodes	X	X	X	X	X
Tests					
Bone scan	X				
CT scan, no contrast axial and coronal cuts	X				
DNA testing	X				
OPHTHALMOLOGIST					
Exam under anesthesia	X	X	X	X	X

Genetic Counseling for Family Members of Index Patient Assuming 80% Penetrance

Family History	Risk Assessment of the Offspring of:
None, unilateral disease	parent—1%
	patient—8%
	sibling—1%
Positive, one or more relatives have tumor, unilateral disease	parent—40%
	patient—40%
	sibling—7%
None, bilateral disease	parent—6%
	patient—40%
	sibling—<1%
Positive, bilateral disease	parent—40%
	patient—40%

Comments: Prognosis depends on the degree of differentiation and stage of tumor, optic nerve involvement, and involvement of the uvea, the vascular tunic of the eye. Overall survival rate is greater than 90% in the United States. RB accounts for 1% of childhood tumor deaths. Enucleation is often the treatment of choice because the tumor usually presents as a large growth. However, eyes are saved that are diagnosed early. The salvage rate approaches 95% in eyes with a lesion less than 4 optic nerve diameters in size.

INTRAOCULAR MELANOMA

CONSULTANTS: Peter E. Liggett, M.D.—Ophthalmic Surgeon
Jonathan E. Sears, M.D.—Ophthalmic Surgeon

The most common primary intraocular malignancy in adult Caucasians. Uveal melanoma accounts for 12% of all melanomas. It occurs eight times more often in whites than in blacks; patients are usually middle-aged or older. Roughly half of patients with uveal melanoma die from metastatic disease within 10 to 15 years after diagnosis and enucleation.

INCIDENCE AND SURVIVAL

	Total	Male	Female
Incidence rate per 100,000/yr	0.7	0.8	0.6
Mortality rate per 100,000/yr	0.1	0.1	0.1
5-year survival rate	77.2%	77.7%	76.6%
10-year survival rate	52%		
15-year survival rate	46%		

Trends

Incidence has been stable for many years in contrast to cutaneous melanoma, which is increasing rapidly. The factors that determine prognosis of uveal melanoma include size, histologic cell type, and secondary glaucoma.

Major risk factors

Exposure to sunlight. Occasional familial occurrence. Rarely associated with cutaneous melanoma.

Pathology

Cell types of uveal melanomas can be described by a modified Callender classification along with their propensity to metastasize: spindle A (17%), spindle B (24%), spindle A and B mixed (29%), predominantly spindle with few epithelioid cells (31%), predominantly epithelioid with or without spindle cells (43%). Pigmentation can be none (amelanotic), mild, moderate, or heavy.

Metastatic sites (major)

May occur as early as 2–4 years or more than 30 years after initial diagnosis, but median is 7 years. The site of metastasis for patients with initial and subsequent involvement of other organs is liver 45/25%, lung 17/23%, subcutaneous tissue and skin 9/26%, lymph nodes 9/6%, GI 3/12%, bone 3/12%, brain 3/3%, and other 9/12%. One percent of patients present with simultaneous uveal and metastatic disease. The association of glaucoma as a preoperative predictor of spread has a predictive positive value of 53%. Nineteen percent of patients without glaucoma demonstrated metastases.

Therapy

Surgery (enucleation or local resection), radiation (external beam or brachytherapy), phototherapy, and diathermy.

Recommendations to patient

Avoid excess ultraviolet light (sunlight and tanning salons).

Recommendations to family

In the rare familial case, genetic counseling may be helpful.

FOLLOW-UP OF THE PATIENT WITH INTRAOCULAR MELANOMA

	1st–10th Year (Months)			Thereafter (Months)
	4	8	12	12

History

Complete	Every 8 months			Every 8 months

Physical

Complete	Every 8 months			Every 8 months
Skin		×		×
Lymph nodes		×		×
Chest		×		×
Abdomen (liver)		×		×

Tests

Chest x-ray	Every 8 months			Every 8 months
CT scan with IV contrast		×		×
Bilirubin, alk phos	×	×	×	Every 8 months
SGOT, SGPT	×	×	×	Every 8 months

Comments: With regard to tumor size, it is often accepted that tumors less than 10 mm in diameter and less than 1.7 mm in height can be observed closely and treated only when enlargement can be documented. Tumors with the largest tumor dimension less than 10 mm have metastases in 19% of patients; this figure rises to 30% in the 10–15-mm range and 70% in the greater than 15-mm largest tumor dimension. Survival rate is stage dependent. Five-year survival is in the range of 70–80% for enucleation and radiotherapy. The desire for the preservation of ocular function has led to the randomized therapies under long-term COMS (Collaborative Ocular Melanoma Study). Five-year mortalilty rates of 20% for charged particle irradiation and 30% for enucleation (50% at 10 years) point out the aggressive metastatic potential of larger tumors.

3 HEAD AND NECK CANCERS

LIP CANCER

CONSULTANT: *Robert M. Byers, M.D.—Otolaryngologist*

Easily confused by the patient with a benign condition, this easily curable cancer can be devastating and fatal if neglected.

INCIDENCE AND SURVIVAL

	Total	Male	Female
Incidence rate per 100,000/yr	1.2	2.4	0.3
Mortality rate per 100,000/yr	0.0	0.1	0.0
5-year relative survival rate	94.1%	94.1%	94.0%
New cancer cases (ACS est 1995)	2500	1900	600
Cancer deaths (ACS est 1995)	100	80	20
5-year relative survival rates by stage			
Stage I	90%		
Stage II	70–80%		
Stage III	50%		
Stage IV	25–50%		

Trends
Earlier diagnosis and awareness of consequences of actinic exposure are reducing incidence.

Major risk factors
Tobacco smoking (including pipes and cigars) and chewing. Actinic exposure (sun's rays, especially ultraviolet bands A and B).

Pathology (major types)
Squamous cell carcinoma.

Metastatic sites (major)
Submandibular and submental lymph nodes. Upper lip lesions may metastasize to periparotid nodes (ie, preauricular nodes) as well as submandibular. Perineural invasion is a poor prognostic sign.

Associated malignancies
Skin, especially cutaneous melanoma.

Therapy
Surgery (primary closure if defect is less than one third of lip), and occasionally radiation.

Recommendations to patient
Avoid smoking tobacco, including pipes and cigars. Reduce sun exposure and tanning studios. Consider use of isotretinoin for 1 year.

FOLLOW-UP OF THE PATIENT WITH LIP CANCER

	1st Year (Months)				2nd Year (Months)			3rd Year (Months)		Thereafter (Months)
	3	6	9	12	4	8	12	6	12	12
History										
Complete				×			×		×	×
Head and neck	×	×	×	×	×	×	×	×	×	×
Physical										
Complete				×			×		×	×
Head and neck	×	×	×	×	×	×	×	×	×	×
Tests										
Chest x-ray				×			×		×	×

Points to Remember: The Rule of 9's

1. 90% occurs in Caucasians.
2. 90% occurs in males.
3. 90% occurs on lower lip.
4. 90% are squamous cancers.
5. 90% do not metastasize.
6. 90% survival.
7. 90% surgical treatment.

ORAL CAVITY CANCER (OC CA)

CONSULTANT: Charles M. Norris, Jr., M.D.—Otolaryngologist

Although most new cases are attributed to use of tobacco (both smoking and chewing tobacco), often in association with alcohol, OC Ca can occur in young adults who do not use tobacco.

INCIDENCE AND SURVIVAL

	Total	Male	Female
Incidence rate per 100,000/yr	6.8	10.9	4.2
Mortality rate per 100,000/yr	2.1	3.3	1.2
New cancer cases (est 1990)	18,200	13,000	5,200
Cancer deaths (est 1990)	5300	3800	1500
5-year relative survival rates by stage			
All stages	52.7%	50.3%	57.8%
Localized	77.7%	77.0%	79.0%
Regional	41.7%	39.5%	46.4%
Distant	19.1%	16.1%	27.0%
Unstaged	43.4%	39.1%	51.6%

Trends

Decreasing incidence in white men, but rising incidence in black men. Overall decrease in both incidence and mortality.

Major risk factors

Tobacco smoking and alcohol ingestion cause 75% of all cases. Smokeless tobacco (particularly snuff) accounts for the large majority of tumors that occur in the cheek and gums. Herpes simplex virus type 1 appears to play a role in etiology.

Pathology (major types)

Squamous cell carcinoma.

Metastatic sites (major)

Lung, adjacent organs, and regional lymph nodes.

Associated malignancies

Lung, other aerodigestive organs, liver, esophagus, and bladder.

Therapy

Surgery, radiation, chemotherapy, and retinoids.

Recommendations to patient

Avoid smoking and chewing tobacco. Consider use of isotretinoin (13-cis-retinoic acid) orally for 1 year.

Recommendations to family

Avoid smoking and chewing tobacco and drinking alcohol.

FOLLOW-UP OF THE PATIENT WITH ORAL CAVITY CANCER

	1st Year (Months)									2nd Year (Months)						3rd Year (Months)				4th Year (Months)			Thereafter (Months)	
	1	2	3	4	5	6	8	10	12	2	4	6	8	10	12	3	6	9	12	4	8	12	6	12
History																								
Complete								X						X				X			X			X
Pain, focal	X	X	X	X	X	X	X	X	X	X	X	X	X	X	X	X	X	X	X	X	X	X	X	X
Dysarthria	X	X	X	X	X	X	X	X	X	X	X	X	X	X	X	X	X	X	X	X	X	X	X	X
Dysphagia	X	X	X	X	X	X	X	X	X	X	X	X	X	X	X	X	X	X	X	X	X	X	X	X
Oral bleeding	X	X	X	X	X	X	X	X	X	X	X	X	X	X	X	X	X	X	X	X	X	X	X	X
Ulceration	X	X	X	X	X	X	X	X	X	X	X	X	X	X	X	X	X	X	X	X	X	X	X	X
Growth	X	X	X	X	X	X	X	X	X	X	X	X	X	X	X	X	X	X	X	X	X	X	X	X
Otalgia	X	X	X	X	X	X	X	X	X	X	X	X	X	X	X	X	X	X	X	X	X	X	X	X
Dental Sx's	X	X	X	X	X	X	X	X	X	X	X	X	X	X	X	X	X	X	X	X	X	X	X	X
Odynophagia	X	X	X	X	X	X	X	X	X	X	X	X	X	X	X	X	X	X	X	X	X	X	X	X
Neck mass	X	X	X	X	X	X	X	X	X	X	X	X	X	X	X	X	X	X	X	X	X	X	X	X
Weight loss	X	X	X	X	X	X	X	X	X	X	X	X	X	X	X	X	X	X	X	X	X	X	X	X
Physical																								
Complete								X						X				X			X			X
Oral	X	X	X	X	X	X	X	X	X	X	X	X	X	X	X	X	X	X	X	X	X	X	X	X
Pharynx	X	X	X	X	X	X	X	X	X	X	X	X	X	X	X	X	X	X	X	X	X	X	X	X
Larynx	X	X	X	X	X	X	X	X	X	X	X	X	X	X	X	X	X	X	X	X	X	X	X	X
Cervical nodes	X	X	X	X	X	X	X	X	X	X	X	X	X	X	X	X	X	X	X	X	X	X	X	X
Dental				X			X		X		X		X		X		X		X	X		X	X	X
Tests																								
Chest x-ray						X			X			X			X		X		X			X		X
Office biopsy	As indicated																							
Operative endoscopy	As indicated																							
Contrast radiography	As indicated																							
Cross-sectional imaging (CT; MRI)	As indicated																							

Comments: While most treatment failures of a squamous cell carcinoma of the upper aerodigestive tract will occur during the first 3 years of follow-up, subsequent second primary cancers are a common enough (10–30%) problem to warrant lifetime surveillance. Patients previously treated for an OC Ca are particularly prone to second OC cancer sites. Given the diversity of mucosal trauma to which the oral cavity is exposed and its proclivity for leukoplakia and premalignant lesions, strategies for prevention, including cessation of tobacco intake and the use of systemic retinoid compounds, are important. It is paramount to eliminate causes of symptomatic ambiguity, for instance, due to dental disease, candidiasis, or xerostomia, in such patients, as well as potential ambiguities in mucosal appearance. Palpation and a low threshold for follow-up biopsy are important adjuncts in surveillance management. Consistency in follow-up is critical in order that the subtle changes that could evolve into a recurrence or second primary lesion be evaluable. Both patient and examiner must adjust to and allow for changes expected due to antecedent treatment (radiation and/or surgery) or ongoing environmental influences (eg, dentures). As in other head and neck sites, metastasis to distant locations outside of the evaluable upper aerodigestive tract (lung, bone, liver) can occur and require forms of evaluation other than history and physical examination.

OROPHARYNGEAL CANCER

CONSULTANT: *Nicholas J. Cassisi, M.D.—Otolaryngologist*

These are aggressive tumors that grow rapidly, are best seen with thorough examinations, are often misdiagnosed, and are generally treated with combined therapy.

INCIDENCE AND SURVIVAL

	Total	Male	Female
Incidence rate per 100,000/yr	0.3	0.5	0.2
Mortality rate per 100,000/yr	0.2	0.3	0.1
5-year relative survival rate	23.4%	19.3%	32.4%
New cancer cases (est 1990)	850	600	250
Cancer deaths (est 1990)	500	360	140
5-year relative survival rates by stage			
Stage I	60–70%		
Stage II	50%		
Stage III	20–30%		
Stage IV	14–20%		

Trends

Earlier diagnosis is the only way at present to improve survival and may be possible with recent progress in diagnostic imaging. High incidence of second primaries.

Major risk factors

Tobacco smoking and chewing, ingesting alcohol, poor oral hygiene, mechanical irritation, Plummer-Vinson syndrome, poor diet.

Pathology (major types)

Squamous cell carcinoma, adenoid cystic carcinoma, and adenocarcinoma.

Metastatic sites (major)

Regional lymph nodes and lung.

Associated malignancies

Other aerodigestive organs, esophagus, lung, and liver.

Therapy

Surgery, radiation, and chemotherapy.

Recommendations to patient

Avoid smoking and chewing tobacco and drinking alcohol.

FOLLOW-UP OF THE PATIENT WITH OROPHARYNGEAL CANCER

	1st Year (Months)								2nd Year (Months)						3rd Year (Months)				Thereafter (Months)	
	1	2	3	4	6	8	10	12	2	4	6	8	10	12	3	6	9	12	6	12
History																				
Complete								X						X				X		X
Pain	X	X	X	X	X	X	X		X	X	X	X	X		X	X	X			X
Dysphagia	X	X	X	X	X	X	X		X	X	X	X	X		X	X	X			X
Odynophagia	X	X	X	X	X	X	X		X	X	X	X	X		X	X	X			X
Neck lump	X	X	X	X	X	X	X		X	X	X	X	X		X	X	X			X
Hoarseness	X	X	X	X	X	X	X		X	X	X	X	X		X	X	X			X
Hemoptysis	X	X	X	X	X	X	X		X	X	X	X	X		X	X	X			X
Physical																				
Complete								X						X				X		X
Oral cavity	X	X	X	X	X	X	X		X	X	X	X	X		X	X	X			X
Pharynx	X	X	X	X	X	X	X		X	X	X	X	X		X	X	X			X
Larynx, indirect	X	X	X	X	X	X	X		X	X	X	X	X		X	X	X			X
Cervical nodes	X	X	X	X	X	X	X		X	X	X	X	X		X	X	X			X
Tests																				
Chest x-ray								X						X				X		X
CT scan	As indicated																			
Barium swallow	As indicated																			

Comments: Although 5-year follow-up has traditionally been used as the standard for upper aerodigestive tract squamous carcinoma, about 95% of treatment failures will occur within 3 years. Metachronous second primary cancers occur in up to one-third of cases, the majority occurring in other head and neck primary sites, the lung, or the esophagus. For this reason, it is important that these patients be followed indefinitely.

NASOPHARYNGEAL CANCER
CONSULTANT: Willard E. Fee, Jr., M.D.—Otolaryngologist

An unusual area for tumors that are somewhat different than most of the other head and neck tumors with a greater diversity of histologic types and the special situation of tumor associated with the Epstein-Barr virus.

INCIDENCE AND SURVIVAL

	Total	Male	Female
Incidence rate per 100,000/yr	0.6	0.9	0.4
Mortality rate per 100,000/yr	0.3	0.4	0.2
5-year relative survival rate	47.3%	44.1%	53.6%
New cancer cases (est 1990)	1550	1050	500
Cancer deaths (est 1990)	730	480	250
5- and 10-yr relative survival rates by stage	No. patients	5 yr (%)	10 yr (%)
Stage I	35	51	34
Stage II	585	59	40
Stage III	507	41	27
Stage IV	175	24	15

Trends
Now that imaging is better and we are more aware of these tumors, the number of new cases may increase without any substantive change in the disease and its true incidence. Although uncommon in the United States, it is extremely common in China, Hong Kong, Singapore, Malaysia, and Tunisia.

Major risk factors
Epstein-Barr virus exposure (infection or transfection), familial cluster factors, southern China ancestry. Dietary factors, especially the ingestion of salt-cured fish that can release volatile nitrosoamines, poor intake of fresh fruits and vegetables, and domestic smoke from burning wood, grass, and exhaust fumes from the rubber industry.

Pathology (major types)
WHO type I keratinizing squamous cell carcinoma; WHO type II nonkeratinizing carcinoma; WHO type III undifferentiated carcinoma. Other histologies occur with much less frequency, eg, lymphomas, minor salivary gland adenocarcinomas, and sarcomas.

Metastatic sites (major)
Regional lymph nodes, adjacent structures (base of the skull, cranial nerves), CNS, lungs, liver, and bone.

Associated malignancies
In patients with lymphoma of the nasopharynx, about 15% will also have or develop lymphoma of the stomach or small intestine.

Therapy
Radiation with or without chemotherapy, and occasional surgery for recurrences or persistent disease at the primary site and/or neck.

Recommendations to family
Seek genetic counseling if family cluster factors are involved.

FOLLOW-UP OF THE PATIENT WITH NASOPHARYNGEAL CANCER

	1st Year (Months)								2nd Year (Months)						3rd Year (Months)				Thereafter (Months)	
	1	2	3	4	6	8	10	12	2	4	6	8	10	12	3	6	9	12	6	12
History																				
Complete								×						×				×		×
Pain	×	×	×	×	×	×	×		×	×	×	×	×		×	×	×			×
Epistaxis	×	×	×	×	×	×	×		×	×	×	×	×		×	×	×			×
Nasal congestion	×	×	×	×	×	×	×		×	×	×	×	×		×	×	×			×
Neck lump	×	×	×	×	×	×	×		×	×	×	×	×		×	×	×			×
Bone pain	×	×	×	×	×	×	×		×	×	×	×	×		×	×	×			×
Physical																				
Complete								×						×				×		×
Nasopharynx	×	×	×	×	×	×	×	×	×	×	×	×	×	×	×	×	×	×	×	×
Oral cavity	×	×	×	×	×	×	×		×	×	×	×	×		×	×	×			×
Pharynx	×	×	×	×	×	×	×		×	×	×	×	×		×	×	×			×
Larynx	×	×	×	×	×	×	×		×	×	×	×	×		×	×	×			×
Cervical nodes	×	×	×	×	×	×	×		×	×	×	×	×		×	×	×			×
Cranial nerves	×	×	×	×	×	×	×		×	×	×	×	×		×	×	×			×
Tests																				
Liver function					×			×			×			×		×		×	×	×
Chest x-ray								×						×				×		×
MRI scan primary				×		×		×		×		×		×		×		×	×	×
Bone scan	As indicated																			

Comments: Although 5-year follow-up has traditionally been used as the standard for upper aerodigestive tract squamous carcinoma, about 90% of treatment failures will occur within 3 years. Recurrences tend to occur submucosal first; hence, the reason for follow-up MRI scans. Early recurrences in the nasopharynx can be resected with 5-year survivals of 44%.

PARANASAL SINUS AND NASAL CAVITY CANCER
CONSULTANT: *Jeffrey D. Spiro, M.D.—Otolaryngologist*

These tumors are rare in the United States and are seen more frequently in Asia and South Africa.

INCIDENCE AND SURVIVAL

	Total	Male	Female
Incidence rate per 100,000/yr	0.6	0.8	0.5
Mortality rate per 100,000/yr	0.2	0.2	0.1
5-year relative survival rate	52.8%	53.5%	51.8%
New cancer cases (est 1990)	1500	900	600
Cancer deaths (est 1990)	500	300	200
5-year relative survival rates by stage			
Stage I	70–90%		
Stage II	60–80%		
Stage III	25–55%		
Stage IV	10–35%		

Trends
Twice as common in men and seen most frequently in the sixth decade of life.

Major risk factors
Occupational exposure to thorotrast, radium, nickel, chromium, mustard gas, and isopropyl alcohol. Seen in higher incidence in the furniture, textile, boot and shoe industries. Possibly associated with chronic sinusitis.

Pathology (major types)
Squamous cell carcinoma (60–70%), adenoid cystic carcinoma plus adenocarcinoma (15–20%), lymphoma (5%), sarcoma (5–6%), and melanoma (2–5%).

Metastatic sites (major)
Regional lymph nodes and lung.

Local extension or recurrence
Oral cavity, orbit of eye, and anterior cranial fossa.

Associated malignancies
Other aerodigestive organs, esophagus, lung, liver, and bladder.

Therapy
Surgery, radiation, and chemotherapy.

Recommendations to patient
Avoid occupational exposure.

FOLLOW-UP OF THE PATIENT WITH PARANASAL SINUS AND NASAL CAVITY CANCER

	1st Year (Months)	2nd Year (Months)	3rd Year (Months)	Thereafter (Months)
History				
Pain	Monthly	Bimonthly	Every 3 months	Every 6 months
Bleeding	Monthly	Bimonthly	Every 3 months	Every 6 months
Visual changes	Monthly	Bimonthly	Every 3 months	Every 6 months
Facial swelling	Monthly	Bimonthly	Every 3 months	Every 6 months
Facial sensory changes	Monthly	Bimonthly	Every 3 months	Every 6 months
Neck lump	Monthly	Bimonthly	Every 3 months	Every 6 months
Physical				
Oral	Monthly	Bimonthly	Every 3 months	Every 6 months
Nasal/sinus (include endoscopic)	Monthly	Bimonthly	Every 3 months	Every 6 months
Cranial nerves	Monthly	Bimonthly	Every 3 months	Every 6 months
Cervical nodes	Monthly	Bimonthly	Every 3 months	Every 6 months
Tests				
Chest x-ray	Annual			
CT scan, nasal/sinus	As indicated; see Comments			

Comments: Paranasal sinus and nasal cavity cancer encompasses a wide variety of pathology and a number of different anatomic sites. In addition, these tumors are uncommon as a group, and an individual clinician will therefore encounter relatively few patients with this type of cancer. For these reasons, follow-up procedures need to be individualized to some extent. The schedule above is best suited for patients with squamous carcinoma, and is also appropriate for patients with mucoepidermoid carcinoma, sarcoma, and melanoma. Patients with adenoid cystic carcinoma and other salivary-type cancers can be seen less frequently initially, but must be followed regularly for at least 10 years.

Local recurrence is the main cause of treatment failure for this type of cancer. For this reason, the main effort in follow-up is directed to the primary site of origin. Depending on the initial location of the cancer, and the type of treatment employed, this area may or may not be easily accessible to direct examination. The use of either rigid or fiberoptic telescopes may facilitate the examination of the nasal cavity and sinuses, and has the added potential for photodocumentation, which may be helpful in making comparisons between examinations. If the primary tumor was situated adjacent to the skull base, or in an area not readily accessible for direct examination, an annual computed tomography scan is a very useful component of follow-up. A baseline scan performed at the conclusion of treatment may also be helpful in future comparisons.

If detected early, local recurrence of nasal cavity or paranasal sinus cancer may be amenable to further therapy. Regional metastases to cervical lymph nodes are uncommon in this type of cancer, but are associated with a poor prognosis when present. The most common site of distant metastases is the lung, which usually indicates incurable disease. It should be noted, however, that patients with adenoid cystic carcinoma, which has a proclivity for pulmonary metastases, have survived for many years with lung metastases.

HYPOPHARYNGEAL CANCER

CONSULTANTS: Roy B. Sessions, M.D.—Otolaryngologist
Jerome C. Goldstein, M.D.—Otolaryngologist

Hypopharyngeal cancer comprises 5–10% of all head and neck cancers.

INCIDENCE AND SURVIVAL

	Total	Male	Female
Incidence rate per 100,000/yr	1.0	1.7	0.4
Mortality rate per 100,000/yr	0.2	0.4	0.1
5-year relative survival rate	24.1%	22.3%	30.0%
New cancer cases (est 1990)	2500	2000	500
Cancer deaths (est 1990)	600	475	125
5-year relative survival rates by stage			
Stage I	50–80%		
Stage II	50–60%		
Stage III*	30–50%		
Stage IV	15–25%		

*Any patient with cervical metastasis is automatically categorized as a stage III or higher; the most significant compromise in survival is generated by cervical metastasis.

Trends

Prognosis is worse for hypopharyngeal cancer than for other pharyngeal cancers.

Major risk factors

Tobacco (smoking or smokeless), alcohol, nutritional deficiencies (Plummer-Vinson syndrome).

Pathology (major types)

Squamous cell carcinoma almost exclusively; adenocarcinoma rarely.

Metastatic sites (major)

Local extension into adjacent cervical spaces, or into laryngeal cartilage. Primary propensity for skip metastasis from one mucosal site to another. Regional metastasis to upper and mid-cervical jugular lymph nodes (over 75% of patients present with cervical metastasis). Distant metastasis to lungs and skeleton.

Associated malignancies

Associated with multiple synchronous primary cancers in 10–20% of cases. Metachronous second primary cancers usually in pharynx, esophagus, or lung.

Therapy

Surgery, radiation, and chemotherapy.

Recommendations to patient

Avoid using tobacco. Avoid nutritional compromise. Avoid alcohol. Follow-up for secondary primary cancers.

Recommendations to family

Avoid tobacco and follow moderate to nondrinking lifestyle. Obtain genetic counseling if familial predisposition is suspected.

FOLLOW-UP OF THE PATIENT WITH HYPOPHARYNGEAL CANCER

	1st Year (Months)							2nd Year (Months)						3rd Year (Months)				Thereafter (Months)	
	1	2	3	4	6	8	10 12	2	4	6	8	10	12	3	6	9	12	6	12
History																			
Complete							X						X				X		X
Pain	X	X	X	X	X	X	X	X	X	X	X	X		X	X	X		X	
Dysphagia	X	X	X	X	X	X	X	X	X	X	X	X		X	X	X		X	
Odynophagia	X	X	X	X	X	X	X	X	X	X	X	X		X	X	X		X	
Hoarseness	X	X	X	X	X	X	X	X	X	X	X	X		X	X	X		X	
Hemoptysis	X	X	X	X	X	X	X	X	X	X	X	X		X	X	X		X	
Neck lump	X	X	X	X	X	X	X	X	X	X	X	X		X	X	X		X	
Physical																			
Complete							X						X				X		X
Oral cavity	X	X	X	X	X	X	X	X	X	X	X	X		X	X	X		X	
Pharynx	X	X	X	X	X	X	X	X	X	X	X	X		X	X	X		X	
Larynx, indirect	X	X	X	X	X	X	X	X	X	X	X	X		X	X	X		X	
Cervical nodes	X	X	X	X	X	X	X	X	X	X	X	X		X	X	X		X	
Tests																			
Chest x-ray							X						X				X		X
CT scan	As indicated																		
Barium swallow							X						X			X			

Comments: Although 5-year follow-up has traditionally been used as the standard for upper aerodigestive tract squamous carcinoma, about 90% of treatment failures will occur within 3 years. Metachronous second primary cancers occur in up to one-third of cases, the majority occurring in other head and neck primary sites, the lung, or the esophagus. For this reason it is important that these patients be followed indefinitely, and that physicians realize that after the initial phase of follow-up, the surveillance is actually for other aerodigestive squamous cancers. If a patient fails to stop smoking and fails to alter drinking habits, these risk factors become substantially higher.

LARYNGEAL CANCER
CONSULTANT: Clarence T. Sasaki, M.D.—Otolaryngologist

The most common cancer of the head and neck and one that is largely preventable.

INCIDENCE AND SURVIVAL

	Total	Male	Female
Incidence rate per 100,000/yr	4.6	8.1	1.7
Mortality rate per 100,000/yr	1.4	2.5	0.5
New cancer cases (ACS est 1994)	12,500	9800	2700
Cancer deaths (ACS est 1994)	3800	3000	800
5-year relative survival rates by stage			
All stages	66.3%	67.8%	60.1%
Localized	84.4%	85.8%	77.1%
Regional	52.9%	53.4%	51.1%
Distant	24.7%	21.1%	36.0%
Unstaged	50.2%	52.1%	41.9%

Trends
Incidence has remained constant over the past two decades. Five-year relative survival rates have also remained stable.

Major risk factors
Tobacco smoking, alcohol ingestion, asbestos, nickel, and mustard gas. Ionizing radiation. Cigarette smokers have nearly a tenfold greater risk than nonsmokers, and the risk rises along with the amount smoked. While heavy alcohol alone is a risk factor, tobacco and alcohol together produce a synergistic effect. Human papilloma virus.

Pathology (major types)
Squamous cell carcinoma, adenocarcinoma, melanoma, neuroendocrine tumors, sarcomas.

Metastatic sites (major)
Lung, adjacent organs.

Associated malignancies
Lung, other aerodigestive organs, liver, esophagus, and bladder.

Therapy
Surgery, radiation, and chemotherapy.

Recommendations to patient and family
Avoid smoking tobacco and drinking alcohol.

FOLLOW-UP OF THE PATIENT WITH LARYNGEAL CANCER

	1st Year (Months)					2nd Year (Months)				3rd–5th Year (Months)		Thereafter (Months)
	1	3	6	9	12	3	6	9	12	6	12	12
History												
Complete					X				X		X	X
Pain	X	X	X	X		X	X	X			X	
Dysphagia	X	X	X	X		X	X	X			X	
Odynophagia	X	X	X	X		X	X	X			X	
Hoarseness	X	X	X	X		X	X	X			X	
Hemoptysis	X	X	X	X		X	X	X			X	
Neck lump	X	X	X	X		X	X	X			X	
Appetite, weight	X	X	X	X		X	X	X			X	
Physical												
Complete					X				X		X	X
Oral	X	X	X	X		X	X	X			X	X
Pharynx	X	X	X	X		X	X	X			X	X
Larynx, indirect	X	X	X	X		X	X	X			X	X
Cervical nodes	X	X	X	X		X	X	X			X	X
Ear	X	X	X	X		X	X	X			X	X
Tests												
Chest x-ray			X		X		X		X		X	X
Barium swallow					X				X		X	
CT scan	As indicated											

Comments: Although 5-year follow-up has traditionally been used as the standard for upper aerodigestive tract squamous carcinoma, about 90% of treatment failures will occur within 2 years; 80% will occur within the first year. Metachronous second primary cancers occur in up to one-third of cases, the majority occurring in other head and neck sites, the esophagus, or the lung. For this reason, it is important that these patients be followed indefinitely.

SALIVARY GLAND CANCER

CONSULTANTS: Jerome C. Goldstein, M.D.—Otolaryngologist
Roy B. Sessions, M.D.—Otolaryngologist

Comprises 3% of all head and neck cancers.

INCIDENCE AND SURVIVAL

	Total	Male	Female
Incidence rate per 100,000/yr	0.9	1.2	0.7
Mortality rate per 100,000/yr	0.2	0.3	0.1
5-year relative survival rate	72.8%	64.9%	81.4%
New cancer cases (est 1990)	2200	1400	800
Cancer deaths (est 1990)	500	360	140
5-year relative survival rates by stage			
Stage I	90%		
Stage II	55%		
Stage III	45%		
Stage IV	10%		

Trends

Prognosis is better in tumors of major salivary glands and worse for minor salivary gland tumors.

Major risk factors

Ionizing radiation and familial predisposition. Wood dust inhalation is associated with the development of adenocarcinoma of the minor salivary glands in the nose and sinuses.

Pathology (major types)

High grade: mucoepidermoid stage III; adenocarcinoma, poorly differentiated; anaplastic carcinoma; squamous cell carcinoma; malignant mixed tumors; adenoid cystic carcinoma. Low grade: acinic cell tumors; mucoepidermoid stages I and II.

Metastatic sites (major)

Lung, adjacent organs, regional lymph nodes, base of the skull, perineural invasion, and especially the facial nerve.

Associated malignancies

Lung, other aerodigestive organs, esophagus, and bladder.

Therapy

Surgery, radiation, and chemotherapy.

Recommendations to patient

Avoid using tobacco. While these tumors are usually slow growing, they need to be followed over a long time period.

Recommendations to family

Avoid using tobacco. Obtain genetic counseling if familial predisposition is suspected.

FOLLOW-UP OF THE PATIENT WITH SALIVARY GLAND CANCER

	1st Year (Months)								2nd Year (Months)						3rd Year (Months)				Thereafter (Months)	
	1	2	3	4	6	8	10	12	2	4	6	8	10	12	3	6	9	12	6	12
History																				
Complete								×						×				×		×
Pain	×	×	×	×	×	×	×		×	×	×	×	×		×	×	×		×	
Dysphagia	×	×	×	×	×	×	×		×	×	×	×	×		×	×	×		×	
Odynophagia	×	×	×	×	×	×	×		×	×	×	×	×		×	×	×		×	
Neck lump	×	×	×	×	×	×	×		×	×	×	×	×		×	×	×		×	
Hoarseness	×	×	×	×	×	×	×		×	×	×	×	×		×	×	×		×	
Hemoptysis	×	×	×	×	×	×	×		×	×	×	×	×		×	×	×		×	
Facial nerve	×	×	×	×	×	×	×		×	×	×	×	×		×	×	×		×	
Physical																				
Complete								×						×				×		×
Oral cavity	×	×	×	×	×	×	×		×	×	×	×	×		×	×	×		×	
Pharynx	×	×	×	×	×	×	×		×	×	×	×	×		×	×	×		×	
Larynx	×	×	×	×	×	×	×		×	×	×	×	×		×	×	×		×	
Cervical nodes	×	×	×	×	×	×	×		×	×	×	×	×		×	×	×		×	
Facial nerve	×	×	×	×	×	×	×		×	×	×	×	×		×	×	×		×	
Tests																				
Chest x-ray								×						×				×		×
CT scan	As indicated																			
Barium swallow	As indicated																			

Comments: Although 5-year follow-up has traditionally been used for upper aerodigestive tract squamous carcinoma, about 95% of treatment failures will occur within 3 years. Metachronous second primary cancers occur in up to one-third of cases, the majority occurring in other head and neck primary sites, the lung, or the esophagus. For this reason, it is important that these patients be followed indefinitely. While most of these tumors are slow growing, there is a subset of mucoepidermoid-type tumors that are aggressive and can grow rapidly, causing local destruction and distant metastases. The adenoid cystic tumors can also metastasize widely, especially to the lungs.

OCCULT PRIMARY METASTATIC (SQUAMOUS CELL) NECK CANCER
CONSULTANT: Barry L. Wenig, M.D.—Otolaryngologist

Represents 5% of all patients with unknown primary carcinoma. In contrast to most patients with adenocarcinoma of unknown primary, patients with squamous cell carcinoma of upper and mid-cervical lymph nodes have a longer survival and occasional long-term freedom from disease recurrence.

Occurrence

Most often seen when upper or middle cervical lymph nodes are involved and indicates a probable primary malignancy in the nasopharynx, base of the tongue, or tonsil. Low cervical or supraclavicular lymph node involvement is more likely associated with a primary neoplasm of the lung, breast, esophagus, or an infradiaphragmatic organ (usually genitourinary).

SURVIVAL	Total	
3-year NED survival rates		
N1	40–50%	(Metastasis in single ipsilateral node 3 cm or less in greatest diameter)
N2	38%	(Metastasis in single ipsilateral node >3 cm but <6 cm)
N3	26%	(Metastasis in node >6 cm)

Trends

Patients who later develop an identifiable primary lesion have a worse prognosis than those whose primary lesion remains occult.

Major risk factors

Tobacco smoking and alcohol abuse.

Pathology (major types)

Squamous cell carcinoma.

Metastatic sites (major)

Lung, liver, and bone.

Associated malignancies

Aerodigestive organs, esophagus, lung, liver, and bladder.

Therapy

Surgery, radiation, and chemotherapy.

Recommendations to patient and family

Avoid smoking tobacco and drinking alcohol.

FOLLOW-UP OF THE PATIENT WITH OCCULT PRIMARY METASTATIC (SQUAMOUS CELL) NECK CANCER

	1st Year (Months)							2nd Year (Months)						3rd Year (Months)				Thereafter (Months)	
	1	2	3	4	6	8	10	12	2	4	6	8	10	12	3	6	9	12	6	12
History																				
Complete								✕						✕				✕		✕
Pain	✕	✕	✕	✕	✕	✕	✕		✕	✕	✕	✕	✕		✕	✕	✕		✕	
Dysphagia	✕	✕	✕	✕	✕	✕	✕		✕	✕	✕	✕	✕		✕	✕	✕		✕	
Odynophagia	✕	✕	✕	✕	✕	✕	✕		✕	✕	✕	✕	✕		✕	✕	✕		✕	
Neck lump	✕	✕	✕	✕	✕	✕	✕		✕	✕	✕	✕	✕		✕	✕	✕		✕	
Hoarseness	✕	✕	✕	✕	✕	✕	✕		✕	✕	✕	✕	✕		✕	✕	✕		✕	
Hemoptysis	✕	✕	✕	✕	✕	✕	✕		✕	✕	✕	✕	✕		✕	✕	✕		✕	
Physical																				
Complete								✕						✕				✕		✕
Oral cavity	✕	✕	✕	✕	✕	✕	✕		✕	✕	✕	✕	✕		✕	✕	✕		✕	
Pharynx	✕	✕	✕	✕	✕	✕	✕		✕	✕	✕	✕	✕		✕	✕	✕		✕	
Larynx	✕	✕	✕	✕	✕	✕	✕		✕	✕	✕	✕	✕		✕	✕	✕		✕	
Cervical nodes	✕	✕	✕	✕	✕	✕	✕		✕	✕	✕	✕	✕		✕	✕	✕		✕	
Tests																				
Chest x-ray								✕						✕				✕		✕
CT scan								✕						✕				✕		✕

Comments: Although 5-year follow-up has traditionally been used as the standard for upper aerodigestive tract squamous carcinoma, about 95% of treatment failures will occur within 3 years. Metachronous second primary cancers occur in up to one-third of cases, the majority occurring in other head and neck primary sites, the lung, or the esophagus. The patients with unknown primary squamous cell carcinoma have about the same survival as patients with head and neck carcinomas of known primary sites. Indeed, some have very prolonged survivals and occasional cures. Hence, follow-up should be prolonged and recurrences can sometimes be retreated successfully for palliation and further extended survival.

4

NON–SMALL-CELL LUNG CANCER (NSCLC)

CONSULTANT: Steven M. Grunberg, M.D.—Medical Oncologist

Lung cancer is the second most common malignancy in the United States (recently exceeded by prostate cancer) but is still the most common cause of cancer death in the country. In 1995 there will be approximately 169,900 new lung cancer cases (96,000 males and 73,900 females) and approximately 157,400 lung cancer deaths (95,400 males and 62,000 females according to ACS estimates). NSCLC accounts for 82% (in some surveys) of all primary lung cancer in the United States.

INCIDENCE AND SURVIVAL

	Total	Male	Female
Incidence rate per 100,000/yr (NSCLC)	48.0	69.9	1.8
New NSCLC cases (est 1995)	139,300	78,700	60,600
5-year relative survival rates by stage (NSCLC)			
Stage I	50%		
Stage II	30%		
Stage III A	10–15%		
Stage III B	<5%		
Stage IV	<2%		

Trends

Some increase in survival. For men, stable incidence and mortality rates. Incidence and mortality rates in women are still increasing.

Major risk factors

Cigarette smoking is the principal cause (85%+) and the risk of dying from lung cancer is 22 times greater among men and 12 times greater among women who smoke compared with nonsmokers. There is also a measurable risk from passive (environmental) smoke. Radon gas can cause lung cancer in concentrations found in mines, but whether concentrations detected in ordinary homes pose a significant risk is still under study. Other agents posing a risk include asbestos (which has a synergistic effect with tobacco smoke), arsenic, chromium, nickel, mustard gas, chloromethyl ethers, and radiation.

Pathology (major types)

Squamous cell (epidermoid) carcinoma, adenocarcinoma, large-cell carcinoma. Incidence of squamous cell is decreasing and adenocarcinoma is increasing.

Metastatic sites (major)

Brain, liver, other lung, bone, adrenal, and skin.

Associated malignancies

Larynx, oral cavity, bladder, pancreas, and esophagus.

Therapy

Surgery, radiation, and chemotherapy.

Recommendations to patient and family

Do not smoke or allow others to smoke near you.

FOLLOW-UP OF THE PATIENT WITH NON–SMALL-CELL LUNG CANCER

	First Year (Months)						2nd–5th Year (Months)				Thereafter (Months)
	2	4	6	8	10	12	3	6	9	12	12
History											
Complete						×				×	×
Cough, dyspnea	×	×	×	×	×		×	×	×		
Chest pain	×	×	×	×	×		×	×	×		
Appetite, weight	×	×	×	×	×		×	×	×		
Hemoptysis, wheezing	×	×	×	×	×		×	×	×		
CNS symptoms	×	×	×	×	×		×	×	×		
Hoarseness	×	×	×	×	×		×	×	×		
Abdominal pain	×	×	×	×	×		×	×	×		
Musculoskeletal pain	×	×	×	×	×		×	×	×		
Physical											
Complete						×				×	×
Lungs	×	×	×	×	×		×	×	×		
Lymph nodes	×	×	×	×	×		×	×	×		
Heart	×	×	×	×	×		×	×	×		
Neurologic	×	×	×	×	×		×	×	×		
Liver	×	×	×	×	×		×	×	×		
Musculoskeletal	×	×	×	×	×		×	×	×		
Tests											
Chest x-ray	×	×	×	×	×	×	×	×	×	×	×
CBC	×		×			×		×		×	×
Alk phos, SGOT, bilirubin	×		×			×		×		×	×
Bronchoscopy	As indicated										
Bone or liver scan	As indicated										
CT or MRI of brain	As indicated										

Comments: Lung cancer remains the only major tumor whose incidence can be reduced by more than 90% by a simple modality—avoidance of smoking. Patients who smoke are also at increased risk for cancers of the oropharynx, larynx, esophagus, and bladder. Hence, these areas should be observed also in follow-up of patients with lung cancer. New pain sites should be x-rayed to detect metastases for which palliation may be considered. If the x-ray is negative, then bone pain should be evaluated with a bone scan. Patients who had hypercalcemia as a paraneoplastic syndrome with the initial presentation of their disease (primarily squamous cell carcinoma) should be watched for recurrence of this problem with periodic calcium levels.

SMALL-CELL LUNG CANCER (SCLC)
CONSULTANT: Steven M. Grunberg, M.D.—Medical Oncologist

Lung cancer is the second most common malignancy in the United States (recently exceeded by prostate cancer) but is still the most common cause of cancer death in the country. In 1995 there will be approximately 169,900 new lung cancer cases (96,000 male and 73,900 female) and approximately 157,400 lung cancer deaths (95,400 male and 62,000 female according to ACS estimates). Small-cell lung cancer accounts for 18% (in some surveys) of all primary lung cancer in the United States.

INCIDENCE AND SURVIVAL

	Total	Male	Female
Incidence rate per 100,000/yr (SCLC)	9.7	12.7	7.5
New SCLC cases (est 1995)	30,600	17,300	13,300
Disease-free survival rates (SCLC)	**2 Years (%)**	**5 Years (%)**	
Limited-stage disease	15–30	6.1	
Extensive-stage disease	1–3	<2	

Trends
Increase in survival, but only a slight decrease in mortality associated with improved therapy.

Major risk factors
Cigarette smoking is the principal cause (85%+), and risk of dying from lung cancer is 22 times greater among men and 12 times greater among women who smoke compared to nonsmokers. There is also a measurable risk from passive (environmental) smoke. Radon gas can cause lung cancer in concentrations found in mines, but whether concentrations detected in ordinary homes pose a significant risk is still under study. Other agents posing a risk include asbestos (which has a synergistic effect with tobacco smoke), arsenic, chromium, nickel, mustard gas, chloromethyl ethers, and radiation.

Pathology (major types)
Small-cell carcinoma of lung with cellular classifications of oat cell, intermediate and mixed.

Metastatic sites (major)
Brain, liver, other lung, bone, adrenal, and skin.

Associated malignancies
Larynx, oral cavity, bladder, pancreas, and esophagus.

Therapy
Chemotherapy, radiation, and occasionally surgery.

Recommendations to patient and family
Do not smoke or allow others to smoke near you.

FOLLOW-UP OF THE PATIENT WITH SMALL-CELL LUNG CANCER

	1st Year (Months)						2nd–5th Year (Months)				Thereafter (Months)
	2	4	6	8	10	12	3	6	9	12	12
History											
Complete						×				×	×
Cough, dyspnea	×	×	×	×	×		×	×	×		
Chest pain	×	×	×	×	×		×	×	×		
Appetite, weight	×	×	×	×	×		×	×	×		
Hemoptysis, wheezing	×	×	×	×	×		×	×	×		
CNS symptoms	×	×	×	×	×		×	×	×		
Hoarseness	×	×	×	×	×		×	×	×		
Abdominal pain	×	×	×	×	×		×	×	×		
Musculoskeletal pain	×	×	×	×	×		×	×	×		
Physical											
Complete						×				×	×
Lungs	×	×	×	×	×		×	×	×		
Lymph nodes	×	×	×	×	×		×	×	×		
Heart	×	×	×	×	×		×	×	×		
Neurologic	×	×	×	×	×		×	×	×		
Liver	×	×	×	×	×		×	×	×		
Musculoskeletal	×	×	×	×	×		×	×	×		
Tests											
Chest x-ray	×	×	×	×	×	×	×	×	×	×	×
CBC	×		×			×		×		×	×
Alk phos, SGOT, bilirubin	×		×			×		×		×	×
Bronchoscopy	As indicated										
Bone or liver scan	As indicated										
CT or MRI of brain	As indicated										

Comments: Lung cancer remains the only major tumor whose incidence can be reduced by more than 90% by a simple modality—avoidance of smoking. Patients who smoke are also at increased risk for cancers of the oropharynx, larynx, esophagus, and bladder. Hence, these areas should be observed also in follow-up of patients with lung cancer. New pain sites should be x-rayed to detect metastases for which palliation may be considered. If the x-ray is negative, then bone pain should be evaluated with a bone scan. If the patient initially had evidence of a paraneoplastic syndrome (ectopic ACTH production, syndrome of inappropriate antidiuretic hormone [SIADH]) or the Eaton-Lambert (myasthenic) syndrome, then one must be alert to the possibility of their recurrence during follow-up. A new lung mass appearing more than 4 years after treatment for SCLC is more likely to be a second primary (such as NSCLC) than a recurrence of the original disease.

MALIGNANT THYMOMA
CONSULTANT: Jerry C. Rosenberg, M.D.—Surgeon

The term *thymoma* is generally restricted to neoplasms of the thymic epithelial cells and excludes pure lymphomas of the organ. These are rare tumors that are slow growing and frequently diagnosed by chest x-ray as a screening procedure or as a diagnostic test for some other indication.

INCIDENCE AND SURVIVAL

	Total	
5-year survival rates by Masaoka stage		
Stage I	93%	Totally encapsulated
Stage II	86%	Capsular invasion into fat or pleura
Stage III	70%	Invasion into pericardium, lung
Stage IV A	50%	Pleural or pericardial implants
Stage IV B		Distant lymphogenous or hematogenous metastases
10-year overall survival	64%	

Major risk factors

Ionizing radiation, particularly in childhood, usually for tonsil or adenoid enlargement, or in infancy for status thymolymphaticus, which at one time was thought to be the cause of sudden crib deaths.

Pathology (major types)

Round or oval cells sometimes with a spindle-shaped nucleus. The cells stain positively with keratin and epithelial membrane antigen (EMA), and negatively for leukocyte common antigen (LCA). Other thymic tumors include lymphomas, Hodgkin's disease, germ cell tumors, carcinoids, and carcinomas.

Metastatic sites (major)

Regional lymph nodes, liver, lung, bone, pleura, and pericardium.

Associated malignancies

Leukemias, lymphomas, Kaposi's sarcoma, other solid tumors including nasopharyngeal carcinoma.

Associated disorders

Myasthenia gravis, red cell aplasia, hypogammaglobulinemia, collagen diseases, Sjögren's syndrome, pemphigus, Eaton-Lambert syndrome, nephrotic syndrome, endocrine disorders, and malignancy involving other organs.

Therapy

Surgery, radiation, and chemotherapy.

Recommendations to patient

Report infection early to physician because of impaired immune function.

Recommendations to family

Obtain genetic counseling if hereditary influence is involved.

FOLLOW-UP OF THE PATIENT WITH MALIGNANT THYMOMA

	1st Year (Months)		2nd–5th Year (Months)		Thereafter (Months)
	6	12	6	12	12
History					
Complete		×		×	×
Cough	×		×		
Hoarseness	×		×		
Lumps	×		×		
Bone pain	×		×		
Muscle spasm	×		×		
Physical					
Complete		×		×	×
Operative site	×		×		
Neck	×		×		
Chest	×		×		
Abdomen	×		×		
Tests					
Chest x-ray	×	×		×	×
CT of chest		×		×	×
CBC	×	×		×	×

Comments: Prognosis for patients with thymoma (all should be considered as malignant tumors) is closely related to the stage of disease at the time of treatment. When the tumor does recur, it is most often a local recurrence. Distal spread is possible but infrequent. Therefore, follow-up examinations should include chest x-ray and CT scans of the chest on a yearly or biannual schedule. Thymomas are very slow growing and cause symptoms by virtue of their size and location in the chest. However, as important as the recurrences are the symptoms that may occur in patients with conditions that are frequently present in those with thymoma. These vary from malignancies at other sites to autoimmune disorders. They can cause as much, or more, morbidity and mortality in patients with thymoma as the tumor itself.

MALIGNANT MESOTHELIOMA
CONSULTANT: Harvey I. Pass, M.D.—Surgeon

Largely a disease of technological civilization that mines, mills, and uses asbestos in construction and industry. About 28 million people in the United States have been exposed occupationally over the last 50 years. Many public buildings and schools contain asbestos, which is being removed at great cost. Whether it could just be covered safely and more economically is a point of great public and political debate.

INCIDENCE AND SURVIVAL

	Total	Male	Female
Incidence rate per 100,000/yr	1.2		
2-year survival rate	32–48%		
4-year survival rate	0–17%		
New cancer cases (est US)	2200	1750	450
Cancer deaths	2000	1600	400

Trends
Incidence increasing.

Major risk factors
Asbestos. Ionizing radiation. Male incidence four times that of women and rises with age. About 30–50% have no asbestos exposure. Other fibers like zeolite have been implicated in Turkey and in Oregon. Immunosuppression. Possible genetic factors or viral factors.

Pathology (major types)
Epithelial (50–60%), sarcomatoid, and mixed.

Metastatic sites (major)
Regional lymph nodes, lung, liver, bone, adjacent organs or membranes.

Associated malignancies
Lung cancer.

Therapy
Surgery, radiation, and chemotherapy.

Recommendations to patient
Do not smoke. Although smoking is not synergistic with asbestos for causing mesothelioma, it exerts strong synergy for lung cancer.

Recommendations to family
Members of the household of asbestos workers should be cautious that clothes, shoes, etc, of asbestos workers are left at the plant and workers shower before leaving workplace. Obtain genetic counseling if hereditary influence is involved.

FOLLOW-UP OF THE PATIENT WITH MALIGNANT MESOTHELIOMA

	1st and 2nd Year (Months)					3rd–5th Year (Months)				Thereafter (Months)	
	1	3	6	9	12	3	6	9	12	6	12
History											
Complete					X				X		X
Cough, dyspnea	X	X	X	X		X	X	X		X	
Chest pain, palpitations	X	X	X	X		X	X	X		X	
Appetite, weight	X	X	X	X		X	X	X		X	
CNS symptoms	X	X	X	X		X	X	X		X	
Abdominal fullness	X	X	X	X		X	X	X		X	
Physical											
Complete					X				X		X
Lungs	X	X	X	X		X	X	X		X	
Lymph nodes	X	X	X	X		X	X	X		X	
Previous wounds	X	X	X	X		X	X	X		X	
Heart	X	X	X	X		X	X	X		X	
Neurologic	X	X	X	X		X	X	X		X	
Liver, ascites	X	X	X	X		X	X	X		X	
Tests											
Chest x-ray	X	X	X	X	X	X	X	X	X	X	
CT chest/upper abdomen	X	X	X	X	X	X	X	X	X	X	
CBC/platelet count	X	X	X	X	X	X	X	X	X	X	
Bone scan, head CT	As indicated										
Abdominal ultrasound	As indicated										
Thoracentesis, closed pleural biopsy, video-assisted thoracoscopy with biopsy	As indicated										

Comments: There are no standard therapies for the management of malignant pleural mesothelioma at this time. Survival is very dependent on the volume or bulk of disease with which the patient presents. Patients with disease confined to the parietal pleura without invasion of the chest wall, diaphragm, pericardium, or visceral pleura (stage I A) have the longest survival. Supportive care is associated with survivals of 6–9 months. Surgery alone, either by pleurectomy-decortication or by extrapleural pneumonectomy, can presently be performed with low mortality (4–6%) at centers that concentrate on the disease. Surgery alone, even for the epithelial histology, is not associated with curative results. Hence, present interest centers on maximal debulking surgery and intraoperative or postoperative adjunctive therapies. These patients usually are part of a protocol situation, and documentation of recurrent disease is crucial. If patients have maximal debulking in the nonprotocol situation, without adjunctive therapy, rigorous documentation of recurrence with frequent CT scans is unnecessary and analysis of chest x-rays and symptoms will suffice. Patients with recurrent disease will present with new-onset shortness of breath from recurrent pleural effusion, pericardial effusion, or pulmonary dysfunction from tumor compression. This is usually associated with cough and chest wall pain. Patients can also present with new-onset ascites, whether their mesothelioma was pleural or peritoneal in origin. A complete examination of all previous surgical wounds must be performed to rule out implantation with evident growth. Lymph node examination, with specific attention to the supraclavicular and axillary chains, should lead one to fine-needle aspiration if the lymph nodes are enlarged. Any hint of ascites should be documented by ultrasound with aspiration and cytologic examination.

The CT scan is the gold standard for documenting recurrent disease which, after pleuropneumonectomy, will appear as an irregular growth of the pleural "rind," associated with diaphragmatic blurring, pericardial thickening, and full costophrenic sulci. MRI has little more to offer compared to CT. Patients with neurologic symptoms should have brain CT or MRI to document rare, but possible, metastases. Adrenal metastases are more commonly seen than bone metastases and will appear on CT/MRI. There are no serum markers for mesothelioma. The platelet count, however, is a prognostic factor, with patients having high platelet counts surviving for shorter intervals than those with normal platelet counts.

5

GASTROINTESTINAL CANCERS

ESOPHAGEAL CANCER
CONSULTANT: John C. Marsh, M.D.—Medical Oncologist

Although the incidence in China is 20 times that in the United States, it is still a major problem in this country both in the number of new cases and the fact that the mortality rate approaches the incidence with few cures and poor survival even when the disease is localized.

INCIDENCE AND SURVIVAL

	Total	Male	Female
Incidence rate per 100,000/yr	3.9	6.4	1.9
Mortality rate per 100,000/yr	3.4	5.9	1.5
New cancer cases (ACS est 1994)	11,000	8000	3000
Cancer deaths (ACS est 1994)	10,400	7800	2600
5-year relative survival rates by stage			
All stages	8.5%	8.0%	9.6%
Localized	19.3%	20.0%	18.2%
Regional	6.3%	6.1%	7.0%
Distant	1.8%	1.5%	2.8%
Unstaged	7.2%	7.1%	7.7%

Trends
Both incidence and mortality are still increasing, especially among men. Survival is improving at the 1– and 2–year level with better therapy, but the 5-year survival has not improved. The incidence of lower esophageal cancer is increasing.

Major risk factors
In the United States, alcohol and tobacco account for 80–90% of this cancer. Low socioeconomic status and inadequate diet also contribute. Some cases of lower esophageal cancer arise from Barrett's esophagus. Tylosis (autosomal-dominant inheritance). Plummer-Vinson syndrome.

Pathology (major types)
Squamous cell carcinoma (60%) predominantly in the upper two-thirds of the esophagus and adenocarcinoma (40%) in the lower one third.

Metastatic sites (major)
Regional lymph nodes, liver, lung, pleura, stomach, kidney, peritoneum, adrenal gland, brain, and bone.

Associated malignancies
Larynx, lung, oral cavity, and pharynx.

Therapy
Surgery, radiation, and chemotherapy.

Recommendations to patient
Avoid alcohol and tobacco. Consume soft foods.

Recommendations to family
Obtain genetic counseling if cancer is on hereditary basis. Limit alcohol intake and tobacco usage.

FOLLOW-UP OF THE PATIENT WITH ESOPHAGEAL CANCER

	1st Year (Months)					2nd–5th Year (Months)			Thereafter (Months)	
	1	3	6	9	12	4	8	12	6	12
History										
Complete					×			×		×
Dysphagia	×	×	×	×		×	×		×	
Substernal distress	×	×	×	×		×	×		×	
Appetite, weight	×	×	×	×		×	×		×	
Cough	×	×	×	×		×	×		×	
Hoarseness	×	×	×	×		×	×		×	
Lumps	×	×	×	×		×	×		×	
Bowel function	×	×	×	×		×	×		×	
Physical										
Complete					×			×		×
Lymph nodes	×	×	×	×		×	×		×	
Chest	×	×	×	×		×	×		×	
Abdomen, liver	×	×	×	×		×	×		×	
Nutrition	×	×	×	×		×	×		×	
Tests										
Chest x-ray	×	×	×		×	×	×	×	×	×
CBC	×	×	×	×	×	×	×	×	×	×
Barium swallow		×	×		×			×		×
Stool for occult blood	×	×	×	×	×	×	×	×	×	×
SGOT, alkaline phosphatase			×		×			×		×
Esophagoscopy	As indicated									
CT chest and abdomen	As indicated									

Comments: The old approach of hopelessness associated with esophageal carcinoma is gradually being replaced by a more aggressive diagnostic and therapeutic attack. Imaging techniques are more successful and include the barium swallow with fluoroscopy, x-ray, and cine, and in selected cases, CT scans. Flexible esophagoscopes have made endoscopy simpler and more acceptable to patients. Techniques for surgical resection and reconstruction have improved. With better localization, megavoltage radiation therapy may be directed more precisely with improved responses. Partial remissions from combination chemotherapy are being recorded from multiple centers with increasing frequency. Significant progress is being made on all fronts.

GASTRIC CANCER

CONSULTANT: David P. Kelsen, M.D.—Medical Oncologist

Sixty-five years ago, gastric cancer was the most frequent cause of cancer death in men and the second in women in the United States. Now it is the seventh most common cause of death in the United States and is tied for eleventh place with ovarian cancer in terms of incidence. However, worldwide, it remains the second most common cause of cancer deaths. A significant shift in location has occurred over the last 10–15 years; proximal tumors now make up almost half of all newly diagnosed neoplasms. This increase is most marked in young, white males (ages 35–55).

INCIDENCE AND SURVIVAL

	Total	Male	Female
Incidence rate per 100,000/yr	7.9	11.8	5.0
Mortality rate per 100,000/yr	4.8	7.1	3.2
New cancer cases (ACS est 1994)	24,000	15,000	9000
Cancer deaths (ACS est 1994)	14,000	8400	5600
5-year relative survival rates by stage			
All stages	17.5%	15.7%	20.4%
Localized	56.2%	54.1%	58.7%
Regional	18.7%	16.9%	21.8%
Distant	2.0%	2.1%	1.9%
Unstaged	10.1%	10.7%	9.3%

Trends
Both incidence and mortality have continued to decrease while survival increases for distal tumors (body and antrum). Proximal tumors (cardia and G-E junction) have markedly increased in incidence.

Major risk factors
Helicobacter pylori infection, cigarette and cigar smoking, alcohol, smoked and salted foods, nitrosamines, chronic atrophic gastritis, older age, low socioeconomic status, pernicious anemia, blood group A individuals.

Pathology (major types)
Adenocarcinoma including signet cell type, tubular, papillary, mucinous (colloid), undifferentiated. Carcinoid, lymphoma, leiomyosarcoma.

Metastatic sites (major)
Regional lymph nodes, liver, and peritoneum; less common are ovary (Krukenberg's tumor), lung, bone, brain, kidneys, and adrenals.

Associated malignancies
Colon, rectum, and breast.

Therapy
Surgery for localized disease, radiation, and chemotherapy for more advanced tumor.

Recommendations to patient
Treatment of *Helicobacter pylori* (controversial). Limit intake of smoked fish and meat. Stop smoking and limit alcohol intake.

Recommendations to family
Obtain genetic counseling if hereditary influences are involved.

FOLLOW-UP OF THE PATIENT WITH GASTRIC CANCER

	1st Year (Months)				2nd Year (Months)				3rd and 4th Years (Months)		Thereafter (Months)
	3	6	9	12	3	6	9	12	6	12	12
History											
Complete				×				×		×	×
Appetite, weight	×	×	×		×	×	×		×		
Abdominal pain	×	×	×		×	×	×		×		
Dysphagia	×	×	×		×	×	×		×		
Heartburn	×	×	×		×	×	×		×		
Physical											
Complete				×				×		×	×
Lymph nodes	×	×	×		×	×	×				
Chest	×	×	×		×	×	×				
Abdomen, masses	×	×	×		×	×	×				
Liver	×	×	×		×	×	×				
Rectal				×				×		×	×
Tests											
Chest x-ray				×				×		×	×
CBC	×	×	×	×		×		×	×	×	×
Stool for blood	×	×	×	×		×		×	×	×	×
CEA		×		×		×		×		×	×
Panendoscopy				×				×		×	×
Liver function		×		×		×		×		×	×
CT scan of abdomen		×		×		×		×	×	×	×

Comments: Carcinoma of the stomach is relatively uncommon. Recurrence may be local, mesenteric, or in the liver. Endoscopy is more reliable for gastric carcinomas than is a GI series. Liver function studies are relatively inaccurate compared to a CT scan. If total/distal gastrectomy has been performed, most of those patients will eventually need supplemental IM vitamin B_{12}.

PRIMARY LIVER CANCER AND INTRAHEPATIC BILE DUCT CANCER
CONSULTANT: Thanjavur S. Ravikumar, M.D.—Surgeon

Although relatively rare in the United States, cancer of the liver is one of the leading causes of death in other parts of the world, especially China and South Africa. In the United States, current statistics may overestimate the mortality rate because metastatic cancer of the liver and adenocarcinoma of unknown primary site are sometimes incorrectly reported as (primary) liver cancer instead of the site of the original malignancy.

INCIDENCE AND SURVIVAL

	Total	Male	Female
Incidence rate per 100,000/yr	2.9	4.4	1.7
Mortality rate per 100,000/yr	2.7	3.9	1.7
New cancer cases (ACS est 1994)	16,100	8800	7300
Cancer deaths (ACS est 1994)	13,200	7200	6000
5-year relative survival rates by stage			
All stages	6.0%	3.6%	10.6%
Localized	14.8%	9.5%	24.4%
Regional	6.2%	4.0%	10.6%
Distant	2.3%	1.0%	4.9%
Unstaged	2.7%	1.6%	5.1%

Trends
Both incidence and mortality are still increasing.

Major risk factors
Hepatitis B and hepatitis C viruses, infection, alcohol, aflatoxin, oxymethalone, iron overload in liver, thorotrast, vinyl chloride, arsenic.

Pathology (major types)
Hepatocellular carcinoma, cholangiocarcinoma, angiosarcoma.

Metastatic sites (major)
Lung and bone.

Associated malignancies
Larynx and esophagus.

Therapy
Surgery, radiation, chemotherapy, and regional therapy (including infusion and other interstitial ablative modalities).

Recommendations to patient
Avoid alcohol.

Recommendations to family
Check for hepatitis B and C infection if that was involved in etiology. Check for hemochromatosis (familial) if iron overload was a contributing factor.

FOLLOW-UP OF THE PATIENT WITH PRIMARY LIVER CANCER AND INTRAHEPATIC BILE DUCT CANCER

	1st and 2nd Year (Months)				3rd–5th Year (Months)		Thereafter (Months)
	3	6	9	12	6	12	12
History							
Complete				×		×	×
Jaundice, itching	×	×	×		×		
Nausea, vomiting	×	×	×		×		
Appetite, weight	×	×	×		×		
Abdominal or bony pain	×	×	×		×		
Urine color	×	×	×		×		
Cough, dyspnea	×	×	×		×		
Bowel function	×	×	×		×		
Physical							
Complete				×		×	×
Abdominal mass	×	×	×		×		
Liver	×	×	×		×		
Jaundice	×	×	×		×		
Ascites	×	×	×		×		
Rectal	×	×	×		×		
Lungs	×	×	×		×		
Neck nodes	×	×	×		×		
Tests							
Chest x-ray				×		×	×
CBC	×	×	×	×	×	×	×
Bilirubin, alk phos	×	×	×	×	×	×	×
Alpha-fetoprotein (AFP)*		×		×	×	×	×
CT scan or ultrasound		×		×		×	×

*Only in patients with hepatoma who were demonstrated to have elevated AFP levels at initial diagnosis.

Comments: CT scan is the most sensitive way of detecting recurrence of carcinoma of the liver, gall bladder, or bile ducts. However, ultrasound can be an excellent substitute. If obstructive jaundice is diagnosed by the above tests, additional tests (such as ERCP or percutaneous transhepatic cholangiography) to identify the site of obstruction may be needed. Because biliary obstruction is often an early sign of recurrence, bilirubin and alkaline phosphatase are indicated. They are sensitive and inexpensive studies.

EXTRAHEPATIC BILE DUCT CANCER
CONSULTANT: Roger I. Jenkins, M.D.—Surgeon

An unusual cancer in that even a very small strategically located tumor can be fatal.

INCIDENCE AND SURVIVAL

	Total	Male	Female
Incidence rate per 100,000/yr	1.1	1.4	0.9
Mortality rate per 100,000/yr	0.6	0.8	0.6
5-year relative survival rate	15.3%	14.9%	15.7%
New cancer cases (est 1990)	2700	1600	1100
Cancer deaths (est 1990)	1600	900	700
5-year relative survival rates by stage			
All stages	15%		
Localized	10–20%		
Regional	<5%		
Distant	<5%		

Trends
Both incidence and mortality are decreasing.

Major risk factors
Choledochal cysts, ulcerative colitis, cholangitis. In Southeast Asia, Oriental liver fluke infections are associated with bile duct cancers. Cholecystitis may play a role. Obesity.

Pathology (major types)
Adenocarcinoma and cholangiocarcinoma.

Metastatic sites (major)
Liver and regional lymph nodes.

Associated malignancies
Liver and gallbladder cancer.

Therapy
Surgery, radiation, and chemotherapy.

Recommendations to patient
Follow diet prescribed.

Recommendations to family
Obtain dietary counseling if obesity is a factor.

FOLLOW-UP OF THE PATIENT WITH EXTRAHEPATIC BILE DUCT CANCER

	1st and 2nd Years (Months)				3rd–5th Years (Months)		Thereafter (Months)
	3	6	9	12	6	12	12
History							
Complete				X		X	X
Appetite, weight	X	X	X		X		
Jaundice, itching	X	X	X		X		
Nausea, vomiting	X	X	X		X		
Abdominal pain	X	X	X		X		
Urine color	X	X	X		X		
Bowel function	X	X	X		X		
Physical							
Complete				X		X	X
Abdominal mass	X	X	X		X		
Liver	X	X	X		X		
Jaundice	X	X	X		X		
Ascites	X	X	X		X		
Tests							
Chest x-ray				X		X	X
CBC	X	X	X	X	X	X	X
Bilirubin, alk phos	X	X	X	X	X	X	X
CEA		X		X	X	X	X
CT or U/S abdomen		X		X		X	X

Comments: Resection of biliary tract cancer with curative intent generally entails resection of the extrahepatic biliary tree, resection of contiguous portions of the hepatic parenchyma (central or lobar hepatectomy) with the reestablishment of biliary drainage through one or more anastomoses between proximal intrahepatic bile ducts and a Roux-en-Y limb of intestine. Recurrence of biliary tract cancer follows two major patterns. Less aggressive tumors may present months to years following resection with biliary obstruction secondary to local anastomotic or intraductal recurrence. More aggressive tumors often present with abdominal distention from widespread intra-abdominal peritoneal visceral studding. Flu-like symptoms of cholangitis with fever and chills is often the first sign of local recurrence. Ultrasonography provides the best and most cost-effective tool for identification of newly obstructed bile ducts in the face of a rising alkaline phosphatase and bilirubin level. Differentiation of recurrent bile duct obstruction from recurrent tumor vs. benign stricture formation is often difficult to ascertain even with percutaneous cholangiography. Cholangiography, however, facilitates delineation of the anatomic location of strictures and allows the placement of metallic or plastic stents for the palliative relief of obstructive lesions. Recurrent bouts of cholangitis unresponsive to stricture dilatation are best managed by daily oral doses of suppressive antibiotics in conjunction with a bile thinning agent. The development of intestinal obstruction is an ominous sign usually associated with diffuse peritoneal studding and is rarely amenable to significant long-term palliation.

GALLBLADDER CANCER

CONSULTANTS: Harold J. Wanebo, M.D.—Surgeon
Dan A. Avradopoulos, M.D.—Surgeon

A relatively uncommon but aggressive cancer that is usually diagnosed late, so that survival is poor overall, although results are good with early diagnosis of localized disease.

INCIDENCE AND SURVIVAL

	Total	Male	Female
Incidence rate per 100,000/yr	1.1	0.8	1.4
Mortality rate per 100,000/yr	0.7	0.5	0.9
5-year relative survival rate	14.0%	17.2%	12.8%
New cancer cases (est 1990)	2700	950	1750
Cancer deaths (est 1990)	1700	600	1100
5-year relative survival rates by stage			
All stages	14%		
Localized	80%		
Regional	<5%		
Distant	<5%		

Trends
Both incidence and mortality are still decreasing.

Major risk factors
Chronic cholecystitis, cholecystoenteric fistula, porcelain gallbladder, adenoma, and obesity. Heredity may play a role.

Pathology (major types)
Adenocarcinoma (90–95%), of which 69% are scirrhous, 24% are papillary, and 7% are colloid; small-cell undifferentiated (oat cell) carcinoma (4–6%); squamous cell carcinoma (3%).

Metastatic sites (major)
Liver (specifically segments IV and V), regional lymph nodes including pericholedochal and peripancreatic lymph nodes.

Associated malignancies
Liver.

Therapy
Surgery, radiation, and chemotherapy.

Recommendations to patient
Follow diet prescribed.

Recommendations to family
Obtain genetic counseling if heredity is a factor.

FOLLOW-UP OF THE PATIENT WITH GALLBLADDER CANCER

	1st and 2nd Years (Months)				3rd–5th Years (Months)		Thereafter (Months)
	3	6	9	12	6	12	12
History							
Complete				×		×	×
Abdominal pain	×	×	×		×		
Weight loss	×	×	×		×		
Anorexia	×	×	×		×		
Jaundice	×	×	×		×		
Nausea, vomiting	×	×	×		×		
Urine color	×	×	×		×		
Feces color	×	×	×		×		
Bowel function	×	×	×		×		
Physical							
Complete				×		×	×
Abdominal mass	×	×	×		×		
Hepatomegaly	×	×	×		×		
Jaundice	×	×	×		×		
Ascites	×	×	×		×		
Tests							
Chest x-ray				×		×	×
CBC	×	×	×	×	×	×	×
Bilirubin, alk phos	×	×	×	×	×	×	×
SGOT, SGPT		×		×	×	×	×
CT or U/S of abdomen		×		×		×	×

Comments: Gallbladder carcinoma is the most common malignant lesion of the biliary tract, yet it represents only 5% of all cancers found at autopsy. This malignancy is associated with a dismal prognosis. In one review of nearly 6000 patients, the 5-year survival was 4%. Most of these long-term survivors were diagnosed incidentally by evaluation of the cholecystectomy specimen by the pathologist. About 88% of patients diagnosed will die within a year of diagnosis with a median survival of 6 months. The poor prognosis is, of course, due to the late diagnosis which is invariably made in this disease. Although some authors recommend radical cholecystectomy (which includes lymphadenectomy and wedge resection of the liver bed), only a few long-term survivors have been reported with this procedure, which is associated with significant morbidity and mortality.

In patients who have been resected initially for cure, there is some controversy whether a second resection will improve survival. However, there is some evidence that suggests these patients may be palliated with radiation treatment. In addition, early diagnosis of recurrence may facilitate palliative procedures including endoscopic sphincterotomy and placement of prosthetic stents. CT scan is the most sensitive method of detecting recurrences within the gallbladder bed and pericholedochal lymph nodes, although ultrasound can be an excellent substitute. Early signs of recurrence include biliary obstruction and abdominal pain. Follow-up in our institution is summarized in the above chart.

PANCREATIC CANCER

CONSULTANT: Ephraim S. Casper, M.D.—Medical Oncologist

An insidious malignancy that causes late symptoms and is hard to demonstrate or detect early enough to provide curative therapy or even significant prolongation of life. While it is the tenth most common cause of cancer in the United States, it is the fifth most common cause of cancer death in the country.

INCIDENCE AND SURVIVAL

	Total	Male	Female
Incidence rate per 100,000/yr	9.1	10.6	8.0
Mortality rate per 100,000/yr	8.4	10.0	2.4
New cancer cases (ACS est 1994)	27,000	13,000	14,000
Cancer deaths (ACS est 1994)	25,900	12,400	13,500
5-year relative survival rates by stage			
All stages	3.3%	2.6%	3.9%
Localized	8.2%	4.7%	10.8%
Regional	3.9%	3.8%	4.0%
Distant	1.5%	1.1%	1.8%
Unstaged	5.4%	4.8%	5.9%

Trends

Both incidence and mortality have decreased slightly.

Major risk factors

Cigarette and cigar smoking, occupational exposure (including benzidine, betanapthylamine derivatives, metal dusts).

Pathology (major types)

Mucin-containing duct cell adenocarcinoma (75%), giant-cell carcinoma, adenosquamous, acinar cell, anaplastic carcinoma, colloid adenocarcinoma, papillary cystic carcinoma, cystadenocarcinoma.

Metastatic sites (major)

Regional lymph nodes, liver, lung, and peritoneum.

Associated malignancies

Gallbladder.

Therapy

Surgery, radiation, and chemotherapy.

Recommendations to patient

Check for diabetes mellitus if not already present.

Recommendations to family

Chemotherapy and radiation are toxic and do not significantly prolong life in the vast majority of patients, although sometimes they are of value. There is no standard treatment for this disease and patients ought to seek investigational approaches if they are motivated to confront the disease proactively.

FOLLOW-UP OF THE PATIENT WITH PANCREATIC CANCER

	1st and 2nd Years (Months)				3rd–5th Years (Months)		Thereafter (Months)
	3	6	9	12	6	12	12
History							
Complete				×	×		×
Appetite, weight	×	×	×		×		
Jaundice, itching	×	×	×		×		
Nausea, vomiting	×	×	×		×		
Abdominal pain	×	×	×		×		
Urine color	×	×	×		×		
Bowel function	×	×	×		×		
Diarrhea	×	×	×		×		
Physical							
Complete				×	×		×
Abdominal mass	×	×	×		×		
Liver	×	×	×		×		
Jaundice	×	×	×		×		
Ascites	×	×	×		×		
Rectal	×	×	×		×		
Tests							
Chest x-ray				×		×	×
CBC	×	×	×	×	×	×	×
Liver function	×	×	×	×	×	×	×

Comments: For patients whose disease has been completely resected, and who receive adjuvant chemoradiotherapy, the schedule of follow-up is dependent on the therapeutic course. Following completion of adjuvant therapy, patients are generally followed every 3 months with physical examination, a CBC, and a biochemical profile. CEA and CA 19-9 are not usually helpful and CT scans and ultrasounds are not generally done because of the lack of efficacy of salvage therapies. For a patient with a locally advanced tumor who opts for treatment, the follow-up during therapy is generally monthly during treatment. Following that, the patient should be followed at least every 2 months. It is unlikely that more than 25% of patients who opt for treatment will be alive after 1 year. For the patients with metastatic disease, whether therapy is being administered or not, since median survival is in the range of 3 months, follow-up is generally on a monthly basis and is targeted toward palliation of symptoms. For a patient who chooses comfort measures only, there is no reason for routine testing of blood chemistries or performing repeated radiologic studies. It is extremely important that the patient be kept free of pain with analgesics on a regular schedule, rather than waiting for the pain to recur and then giving pain medication. When narcotics are necessary, they should be given in large enough doses and frequently enough to keep the patient pain-free. They are unlikely to produce addiction if the patient was not previously addicted. Since narcotics are very constipating, liberal but judicious use of laxatives is indicated. When pain control is not successful with narcotics alone, when opiate side effects are unacceptable, percutaneous neurolysis may provide significant relief. Antidepressants and amphetamines may be useful adjuncts to opiate therapy.

SMALL INTESTINE CANCER

CONSULTANT: William F. Sindelar, M.D.—Surgeon

Represents 2% of all alimentary tract cancers and 0.2% of all malignancies in the United States. An uncommon diagnosis, often questioned because of seeming rarity. If within reach of endoscope, the diagnosis may be made preoperatively. If within the jejunum or ileum, the diagnosis may be difficult and may be delayed until disease is advanced.

INCIDENCE AND SURVIVAL

	Total	Male	Female
Incidence rate per 100,000/yr	1.1	1.3	0.8
Mortality rate per 100,000/yr	0.5	0.6	0.4
5-year relative survival rate	45%	43%	49%
New cancer cases (est 1994)	2300	1400	900
Cancer deaths (est 1994)	950	500	450

5-year relative survival rates by stage	By stage	By tumor type
Stage I	75%	Adenocarcinoma 30%
Stage II	50%	Carcinoid 50%
Stage III	25%	Sarcoma 35%
Stage IV	5%	Lymphoma 50%

Trends

Incidence is apparently increasing, probably due to improved diagnosis, endoscopy, and imaging. Mortality is decreasing, probably due to more aggressive treatment.

Major risk factors

Celiac disease, Crohn's disease, von Recklinghausen's disease.

Pathology (major types)	% of small intestinal malignancies	Characteristic distribution
Adenocarcinomas	45%	Most common proximally (45% in duodenum)
Carcinoid	35%	Typically in ileum (90%); can be multicentric (30%)
Sarcoma	15%	Usually leiomyosarcoma; found throughout small intestine
Lymphoma	5%	Most common distally; often associated with extraintestinal disease

Metastatic sites (major)

All types can recur locally. Adenocarcinomas, carcinoids, and lymphomas spread to regional nodes. Adenocarcinomas and carcinoids hematogenously metastasize to liver. Sarcomas metastasize to lung and liver. Lymphomas may be present with systemic disease.

Associated malignancies

Up to 25% of patients with small-bowel cancer have second primary tumors, often but not exclusively gastrointestinal; reason unknown but may be related to immune deficiency and poor immunologic surveillance.

Therapy

Surgery to resect primary. Radiation for locally extensive disease. Chemotherapy for metastatic disease and for lymphomas of all stages.

FOLLOW-UP OF THE PATIENT WITH SMALL INTESTINE CANCER

	1st Year (Months)				2nd Year (Months)				3rd–5th Year (Months)		Thereafter (Months)
	3	6	9	12	3	6	9	12	6	12	12
History											
Complete				X				X		X	X
Appetite, weight	X	X	X		X	X	X		X		
Abdominal pain	X	X	X		X	X	X		X		
Dyspepsia	X	X	X		X	X	X		X		
Nausea, vomiting	X	X	X		X	X	X		X		
Jaundice	X	X	X		X	X	X		X		
Bowel function	X	X	X		X	X	X		X		
Physical											
Complete				X				X		X	X
Lymph nodes	X	X	X		X	X	X		X		
Chest	X	X	X		X	X	X		X		
Abdomen, masses	X	X	X		X	X	X		X		
Liver	X	X	X		X	X	X		X		
Rectal	X	X	X		X	X	X		X		
Tests											
CBC	X	X	X	X	X	X	X	X	X	X	X
Electrolytes	X	X	X	X	X	X	X	X	X	X	X
Liver function	X	X	X	X	X	X	X	X	X	X	X
CEA		X		X		X		X	X	X	X
Stool for blood	X	X	X	X	X	X	X	X	X	X	X
CT scan of abdomen		X		X		X		X	X	X	X
Liver ultrasound*		X		X		X		X	X	X	X
GI endoscopy**		X		X		X		X	X	X	X
GI series/small bowel		X		X		X		X	X	X	X
Chest x-ray		X		X		X		X	X	X	X
5-HIAA***	As indicated										
Bone scan	As indicated										

*If CT scan suspicious or inadequate to evaluate liver.
**For duodenal lesions or locations within reach of endoscope.
***If malignant carcinoid is suspected. See section on gastrointestinal carcinoid.

Comments: Malignancies of the small intestine are rare. Most adenocarcinomas, which after resection can recur locally, leading to ulceration, bleeding, and obstruction, may metastasize to the liver or other distant sites. Carcinoids can recur locally and metastasize principally to the liver. Sarcomas recur locally and metastasize to the liver and lung. Lymphomas typically recur with systemic disease. CT scans are useful for evaluating local recurrences and for hepatic metastasis. Chest x-rays can evaluate for pulmonary metastasis, but chest CT is more sensitive. GI series with small-bowel follow-through may detect locally recurrent disease, but usually is not highly sensitive. GI endoscopy is useful for follow-up of duodenal lesions or other sites within reach of the endoscope.

GASTROINTESTINAL CARCINOID
CONSULTANT: Larry K. Kvols, M.D.—Medical Oncologist

The most common gut endocrine tumor, accounting for 13–34% of all tumors of the small bowel and 17–46% of all malignant tumors of the small bowel. The carcinoid syndrome (flushing, gastrointestinal hypermotility, watery diarrhea, heart disease, bronchial constriction, myopathy) occurs in less than 10% of patients with carcinoid tumors.

INCIDENCE AND SURVIVAL

	Total
Incidence rate per 100,000/yr	1.5
New cancer cases (est 1994)	2500
5-year survival rates by stage	
All stages	82%
Localized	94%
Regional	64%
Distant	18%

Trends

Found in small intestine, pancreas, rectum, ovary, and lung.

Major risk factors

Part of hereditary MEN-I (multiple endocrine neoplasia, type I) syndrome.

Pathology (major types)

Argentaffin tumors with uniform granular cells (Kulchitsky's cells) in nodules or cords.

Metastatic sites (major)

Regional lymph nodes, liver, and bone.

Associated malignancies

Pancreas, adrenal, thyroid, and parathyroid.

Therapy

Surgery, radiation, hormones, chemotherapy, and possibly immunotherapy.

Recommendations to patient

If severe diarrhea and flushing develop, ask physician for symptom therapy.

Recommendations to family

Obtain genetic counseling if hereditary influence is involved.

FOLLOW-UP OF THE PATIENT WITH GASTROINTESTINAL CARCINOID

	1st Year (Months)		Thereafter (Months)
	6	12	12
History			
Complete	×	×	×
Appetite, weight	×	×	×
Abdominal pain	×	×	×
Flushing	×	×	×
Diarrhea	×	×	×
Wheezing	×	×	×
Leg edema	×	×	×
Tachycardia, palpitations	×	×	×
Physical			
Complete	×	×	×
Tests			
Chest x-ray		×	×
CBC	×	×	×
Liver function	×	×	×
24-hour urine 5-HIAA	×	×	×
CT scan of abdomen and pelvis or whole-body somatostatin receptor scintigraphy		×	×

Comments: Carcinoid tumors arising in the gastrointestinal tract or the pancreas most often recur in the liver. Sites of possible recurrence include the mesentery, lymph nodes, peritoneum, and skeleton. Surgery remains the only curative modality, and if isolated metastases are detected, particularly after a long disease-free interval, resection should be considered. The carcinoid syndrome may manifest as flushing, diarrhea, wheezing, or much less frequently, right-sided heart failure. In the vast majority of cases, the development of the carcinoid syndrome will be associated with an increase in the 24-hour urinary excretion of 5-hydroxyindoleacetic acid (5-HIAA). When these symptoms occur and the 24-hour 5-HIAA is elevated, it usually implies hepatic metastases. Loperamide, codeine, or in refractory cases, tincture of opium, is usually helpful in controlling the diarrhea. For patients with significant symptoms related to the flushing or diarrhea that is not responsive to simple medications, a trial of somatostatin analog, octreotide, should be considered. A positive somatostatin receptor scintigram implies that the tumor metastases have receptors for somatostatin and that the patient will respond to octreotide injections. For patients not responding to octreotide or for those who develop refractoriness to the drug, hepatic artery embolization followed by systemic chemotherapy is a useful approach for managing hepatic-dominant metastatic disease. For progressive metastatic disease not confined to the liver, single-agent and combination chemotherapy have limited usefulness. Consideration should be given to referral of the patient for participation in an ongoing trial in that situation.

COLON CANCER

CONSULTANT: *Alfred M. Cohen, M.D.—Surgeon*

The fourth most common malignancy in the United States affecting one in 20 persons and representing 15% of all cancers. Mortality figures are only available for colorectal cancer, although incidence and survival figures are available for colon and rectal cancers separately.

INCIDENCE AND SURVIVAL

	Total	Male	Female
Incidence rate per 100,000/yr	35.0	41.2	30.6
Mortality rate per 100,000/yr (colorectal)	19.4	23.9	16.3
(no mortality data available for colon alone)			
New cancer cases (ACS est 1995)	100,000	49,000	51,000
Cancer deaths (ACS est 1995)	47,500	23,000	24,500
5-year relative survival rates by stage			
All stages	58.8%	59.8%	58.0%
Localized	91.8%	93.7%	90.0%
Regional	60.9%	60.4%	61.3%
Distant	6.1%	6.1%	6.0%
Unstaged	31.0%	34.1%	28.4%

Trends

Mortality has fallen significantly while incidence is still increasing and survival rate has increased. This change is associated with earlier diagnosis and improved treatment results. Cancers are occurring more proximally in the colon and less in the rectosigmoid.

Major risk factors

Diets high in animal fat and meat and low in fiber. Increasing age. Familial polyposis. Familial cancer syndromes. Chronic ulcerative colitis. Granulomatous (Crohn's) colitis. Irradiation of the pelvis and/or abdomen. Previous malignancy of colon or rectum.

Pathology (major types)

Adenocarcinoma accounts for 90–95%, of which the colloid (mucinous) type comprises 17% and the signet-ring cell type comprises 2–4% of those. Scirrhous tumors and carcinoma simplex are rare as are lymphomas and leiomyosarcomas. From 2% to 7% of carcinoids may appear in the colon.

Metastatic sites (major)

Pericolic, intermediate, and principal levels of lymph nodes. Liver, lung, bone, kidney, adrenal, and brain.

Associated malignancies

Uterus, breast, prostate, and ovary.

Therapy

Surgery, radiation, chemotherapy, and immunotherapy.

Recommendations to patient

Increase fiber and vegetables and decrease fat in diet.

Recommendations to family

If question of familial or genetic association, obtain genetic counseling. Yearly digital rectal examination beginning at age 40, stool for occult blood yearly after age 50, and flexible sigmoidoscopy every 3–5 years. If familial disease is suspected, screening should begin much earlier depending on type and current age.

FOLLOW-UP OF THE PATIENT WITH COLON CANCER

	1st–3rd Year (Months)				4th–5th Year (Months)		6th–8th Year (Years)	Thereafter (Years)
	3	6	9	12	6	12	12	12
History								
Interval	×	×	×	×	×	×	×	×
Appetite	×	×	×	×	×	×	×	
Abdominal pain	×	×	×	×	×	×	×	
Bowel function	×	×	×	×	×	×	×	
Physical								
Complete				×		×	×	×
Abdomen	×	×	×	×	×	×	×	
Liver	×	×	×	×	×	×	×	
Scars	×	×	×	×	×	×	×	
Rectal	×	×	×	×	×	×	×	
Prostate (males)				×		×	×	×
Breasts (females)				×		×	×	×
Pelvic (females)				×		×	×	×
Tests								
Stool occult blood	×	×	×	×	×	×	×	×
CBC				×		×	×	
CEA	×	×	×	×	×	×	×	
Colonoscopy				×	then every 3 years			
Chest x-ray				×		×	×	
PSA (males over 50)				×		×	×	×
Mammography (females over 40)				×		×	×	×

Comments: The goals of follow-up are to detect potentially curable recurrences, manage treatment-related dysfunction, early detection of bowel and other organ cancers. Detection of asymptomatic hepatic recurrence is best accomplished by serial CEA determinations. Data suggest this strategy (with subsequent complete evaluation for increasing values) is effective, but not cost-effective. Follow-up visits for the first 3 years may be every 3 or 4 months. Yearly follow-up from 5 to 8 years is important. Lifetime follow-up is essential. In the absence of symptoms, physical findings, or elevated CEA, routine abdominal CT is not indicated.

Rectal Cancer
Consultant: Alfred M. Cohen, M.D.—Surgeon

Although generally grouped with colon cancer as colorectal cancer, rectal cancer has some unique aspects. Nonetheless, mortality statistics are reported only for colorectal cancer, although incidence and survival figures are available for them separately.

INCIDENCE AND SURVIVAL

	Total	Male	Female
Incidence rate per 100,000/yr	14.0	18.6	10.6
Mortality rate per 100,000/yr (colorectal)	19.4	23.9	16.3
(no mortality data available for rectal alone)			
New cancer cases (ACS est 1995)	38,200	21,700	16,500
Cancer deaths (ACS est 1995)	7800	4200	3600
5-year relative survival rates by stage			
All stages	56.3%	55.8%	57.0%
Localized	84.8%	84.7%	85.0%
Regional	51.1%	51.5%	50.5%
Distant	5.1%	4.9%	5.4%
Unstaged	36.9%	38.4%	35.3%

Trends

Mortality has fallen significantly while incidence has also decreased somewhat. Earlier diagnosis and more effective therapy are mainly responsible for improved survival rates.

Major risk factors

Diets high in animal fats and meat and low in fiber. Increasing age. Familial polyposis. Familial cancer syndromes. Chronic ulcerative colitis. Granulomatous (Crohn's) colitis. Irradiation of the pelvis. Previous malignancy of colon or rectum.

Pathology (major types)

Adenocarcinoma accounts for 90–95%, including its subtypes, colloid (mucinous), signet-ring cell, scirrhous, and carcinoma simplex.

Metastatic sites (major)

Pararectal and regional draining lymph nodes. Liver, lung, bone, kidney, adrenal, and brain.

Associated malignancies

Uterus, breast, colon, prostate, and ovary cancer.

Therapy

Surgery, radiation, and chemotherapy.

Recommendations to patient

Increase fiber and vegetables and decrease fat in diet.

Recommendations to family

If question of familial or genetic association, obtain genetic counseling. Yearly digital rectal examination beginning at age 40, stool for occult blood yearly after age 50, and flexible sigmoidoscopy every 3–5 years. If familial disease is suspected, screening should begin much earlier depending on type and current age.

FOLLOW-UP OF THE PATIENT WITH RECTAL CANCER

	1st–3rd Year (Months)				4th –5th Year (Months)		6th–8th Year (Years)	Thereafter (Years)
	3	6	9	12	6	12	12	12
History								
Interval	×	×	×	×	×	×	×	×
Appetite	×	×	×	×	×	×	×	
Abdominal pain	×	×	×	×	×	×	×	
Buttock pain	×	×	×	×	×	×	×	
Perineal pain	×	×	×	×	×	×	×	
Leg pain	×	×	×	×	×	×	×	
Bowel function	×	×	×	×	×	×	×	
Urinary function		×		×	×	×	×	
Sexual function		×		×				
Physical								
Complete				×		×	×	×
Abdomen	×	×	×	×	×	×	×	
Liver	×	×	×	×	×	×	×	
Abdominal scars	×	×	×	×	×	×	×	
Perineal scar (APR)*	×	×	×	×				
Rectal	×	×	×	×	×	×	×	
Prostate (males)				×		×	×	×
Breasts (females)				×		×	×	×
Pelvic (females)	×	×	×	×	×	×	×	×
Inguinal nodes	×	×	×	×	×	×	×	
Tests								
Stool occult blood	×	×	×	×	×	×	×	×
CBC				×		×	×	
CEA	×	×	×	×	×	×	×	
Sigmoidoscopy		×		×	×	×	×	
Colonoscopy				×	then every 3 years			
Chest x-ray				×		×	×	
PSA (males over 50)				×		×	×	×
Mammography (females over 40)				×		×	×	×

*APR=Abdominal-perineal resection.

Comments: See Colon follow-up for comments. Serial sigmoidoscopy and more aggressive pelvic examinations in women are warranted. In the absence of symptoms, physical findings, or elevated CEA, routine and pelvic CT is not indicated.

ANAL CANAL AND ANUS CANCER
CONSULTANT: A. Rahim Moossa, M.D.—Surgeon

Representing 1–3% of all large-bowel cancers and 3.9% of anorectal cancers, it is an uncommon cancer.

INCIDENCE AND SURVIVAL

	Total	Male	Female
Incidence rate per 100,000/yr	0.9	0.8	0.9
Mortality rate per 100,000/yr	0.1	0.1	0.1
5-year relative survival rate	61.7%	57.3%	64.3%
New cancer cases (est 1990)	2200	1000	1200
Cancer deaths (est 1990)	250	120	130
5-year relative survival rates by stage			
Stage I	95%		
Stage II	75%		
Stage III A	60%		
Stage III B	10%		
Stage IV	0.1%		

Trends
Increasing incidence due primarily to young male homosexuals.

Major risk factors
Anal intercourse among young male homosexuals. Condylomata accuminata. Human papilloma virus infection, herpes simplex virus type 1, and *Chlamydia trachomatis* infection. Radiation. Immunosuppression. Cigarette smoking.

Pathology (major types)
Epidermoid (squamous cell) carcinoma (63%), transitional cell (cloacogenic) carcinoma (23%), adenocarcinoma (7%), with remainder comprising basal cell carcinoma, Paget's disease, and melanoma.

Metastatic sites (major)
Abdominal and inguinal lymph nodes, liver, and lung.

Associated malignancies
Cervix, vagina, vulva, and bladder.

Therapy
Surgery, radiation, and chemotherapy.

Recommendations to patient
Avoid smoking tobacco. Avoid unprotected anal intercourse.

Recommendations to family
Avoid smoking tobacco. Observe body fluid infectious precautions.

FOLLOW-UP OF THE PATIENT WITH ANAL CANAL AND ANUS CANCER

	1st Year (Months)				2nd–5th Year (Months)		Thereafter (Months)
	3	6	9	12	6	12	12
History							
Complete				✕	✕		✕
Appetite, weight	✕	✕	✕		✕		
Bowel function	✕	✕	✕		✕		
Abdominal pain	✕	✕	✕		✕		
Jaundice	✕	✕	✕		✕		
Urine color	✕	✕	✕		✕		
Physical							
Complete				✕	✕		✕
Abdomen	✕	✕	✕		✕		
Rectal or stoma	✕	✕	✕		✕		
Jaundice	✕	✕	✕		✕		
Lymph nodes	✕	✕	✕		✕		
Tests							
Chest x-ray				✕		✕	✕
CBC	✕	✕	✕	✕	✕	✕	✕
Stool for blood	✕	✕	✕	✕	✕	✕	✕
Liver function		✕		✕	✕	✕	✕
CT scan of abdomen	As indicated						
Sigmoidoscopy		✕		✕	✕	✕	Every 3 years

Comments: Carcinoma of the anus recurs most frequently locally or with metastases in the abdominal and/or inguinal lymph nodes, the liver, and lung. Pelvic recurrences of anorectal tumors are hard to detect early and sometimes require a CT scan. Liver metastases are also detectable on CT scan. Early, localized tumors are treated with surgical excision. Larger tumors are now more frequently being treated with multimodality therapy with a combination of fluorouracil, mitomycin C, and radiation therapy with sphincter preservation and 75–80% 5-year survival. Patients with metastatic tumors are generally treated empirically with fluorouracil and cisplatin (or other drugs), but should be entered into clinical trials when available to ascertain better methods of therapy.

6

GENITOURINARY CANCERS

RENAL CELL CANCER

CONSULTANT: *Neil H. Bander, M.D.—Urologist*

An adenocarcinoma that arises from the parenchyma of the kidney and accounts for 2.3% of all cancers and 85% of kidney cancers. The average age at presentation, 55 to 60 years, is decreasing as serendipitous early diagnoses are being made by ultrasonography and CT scans performed for other indications. The stage 1 lesions have a high surgical cure rate. Transitional cell carcinoma (TCC) of the renal pelvis and ureter (see page 58) arises from cells lining the collecting system and its behavior is similar to TCC of the bladder and different from renal cell carcinoma (RCC). However, available statistics in regard to incidence, mortality, new cases and cancer deaths, group together RCC and renal pelvis cancer.

INCIDENCE AND SURVIVAL

	Total	Male	Female
Incidence rate per 100,000/yr	8.5	11.8	5.9
Mortality rate per 100,000/yr	3.4	4.9	2.3
New cancer cases (ACS est 1994)	27,600	17,000	10,600
Cancer deaths (ACS est 1994)	11,300	6800	4500
5-year relative survival rates by stage			
All stages	55.3%	56.3%	53.8%
Localized	85.5%	86.4%	84.1%
Regional	56.5%	59.2%	59.1%
Distant	9.5%	10.1%	8.6%
Unstaged	30.3%	29.8%	30.8%

Trends
Both incidence and mortality are increasing.

Major risk factors
Genetic: familial renal cell carcinoma; Lindau–von Hippel disease (tumor suppressor gene on 3p).

Pathology (major types)
Clear cell, granular cell, spindle cell, or sarcomatoid, 85%; papillary, 10%; oncocytomas, 5%.

Metastatic sites (major)
Lung, lymph nodes, bone, liver, adrenal, brain, and spinal cord.

Therapy
Surgery, immunotherapy, and chemotherapy.

Recommendations to family
Consider possible genetic basis in patients who are young and/or who have multifocal and/or bilateral lesions.

FOLLOW-UP OF THE PATIENT WITH RENAL CELL CANCER

	1st Year (Months)				2nd Year (Months)			3rd–4th Year (Months)		Thereafter (Months)
	3	6	9	12	4	8	12	6	12	12
History										
Complete				×		×			×	×
Hematuria	×	×	×		×	×		×		×
Appetite, weight	×	×	×		×	×		×		×
Respiratory symptoms (cough)	×	×	×		×	×		×		×
Back (bone) pain	×	×	×		×	×		×		×
Fever	×	×	×		×	×		×		×
Night sweats	×	×	×		×	×		×		×
Fatigue	×	×	×		×	×		×		×
CNS symptoms	×	×	×		×	×		×		×
Physical										
Complete				×		×			×	×
Abdomen	×	×	×		×	×		×		×
Liver	×	×	×		×	×		×		×
Lymph nodes	×	×	×		×	×		×		×
Chest	×	×	×		×	×		×		×
Tests										
Chest x-ray	×	×	×	×		×			×	Every 2 years
CBC	×	×	×	×	×	×	×		×	Every 2 years
Sonogram and/or CT	As indicated*									
Bone scan	As indicated**									

*Sonogram and/or CT are indicated in the following circumstances: (1) high-stage disease (stage C or D) where recurrence is more likely; (2) for evaluation of new-onset back pain; (3) for examination of contralateral kidney in case of relatively young patient or one with multifocal disease in the resected kidney (where contralateral involvement is more likely).
**Bone scan is indicated to evaluate new-onset bone pain.

Comments: Recurrences of renal cell carcinoma are usually within 3 years, but have been reported as late as 30 years postnephrectomy. While any organ may be a site of recurrence, the most common sites of metastases are lung, lymph node, bone, liver, adrenal, and brain. Local recurrence in the renal bed is rare (approximately 5%), occurs most often in high-stage cancers, and usually presents with back pain. Solitary sites of metastatic disease occur in about 3% of cases and may be curable surgically, particularly if they develop more than 2 years postnephrectomy. Surgery is the only curative modality. Radiotherapy and chemotherapy may be palliative. Hormonal therapy, once the mainstay of treatment for metastatic disease, has been shown to provide no objective benefit. Immunotherapy is beginning to play a role, and interleukin-2 therapy is approved for renal cancer, although the response rate remains quite low and the toxicity is high. A suppressor oncogene located on chromosome 3p is mutated or deleted in virtually all Lindau–von Hippel disease, familial and sporadic cases of clear, granular, or sarcomatoid renal cancer. When this defect is inherited, patients tend to present at a younger age and with multifocal and/or bilateral disease. Even in the absence of a known family history, if a patient presents in such a manner, consideration should be given to screening family members.

TRANSITIONAL CELL CANCER OF RENAL PELVIS AND URETER

CONSULTANT: David Esrig, M.D.—Urologist

Accounts for 7% of all renal tumors and less than 1% of all genitourinary neoplasms. Bladder tumors are 17 times more common.

SURVIVAL

	Total
5-year survival rate by location and stage	
Renal pelvis	
Stages I and II	50–80%
Stages III and IV	0–33%
Ureter	10–20% lower than renal pelvis

Trends

Seen twice as frequently in men. Both incidence and mortality continue to increase.

Major risk factors

Occupational exposure (benzidine, aminophenols, etc), phenacetin abuse, cigarette smoking. Balkan nephropathy is probably familial in patients of Balkan and Greek origin. A kindred of familial transitional cell carcinoma has been reported.

Pathology (major types)

Transitional cell carcinoma (>90%) and squamous cell carcinoma (<10%); adenocarcinoma is rare.

Metastatic sites (major)

Regional lymph nodes, adjacent organs, liver, lung, and bone.

Associated malignancies

Bladder (30–50% incidence in setting of upper-tract malignancy). Contralateral renal pelvis or ureter in 3–4%. Lung, pharynx, and esophagus.

Therapy

Surgery, endoscopic laser ablation, radiation, and chemotherapy.

Recommendations to patient

Avoid tobacco smoking. Avoid occupational chemical exposure when possible.

Recommendations to family

Obtain genetic counseling if involved with familial type of malignancy.

FOLLOW-UP OF THE PATIENT WITH TRANSITIONAL CELL CANCER OF RENAL PELVIS AND URETER

	1st Year (Months)				2nd–5th Year (Months)		Thereafter (Months)
	3	6	9	12	6	12	12
History							
Complete				×		×	×
Hematuria	×	×	×		×		
Bone pain	×	×	×		×		
Physical							
Complete				×		×	×
Abdomen	×	×	×		×		
Rectal	×	×	×		×		
Lymph nodes	×	×	×		×		
Ureteroscopy	×	×		×	×	×	×
Pelvic (female)		×		×	×	×	×
Tests							
Chest x-ray				×		×	×
CBC		×		×		×	×
Urine	×	×	×	×	×	×	×
BUN, alkaline phosphatase		×		×		×	×
IVP		×		×	×	×	×
Urine cytology		×		×		×	×

Comments: Carcinoma of the renal pelvis and ureter is mainly transitional cell carcinoma and its treatment is based on the grade of tumor and its location. Low-grade tumors throughout the renal pelvis and ureter can be treated with endoscopic resection if accessible by the ureteroscope; however, surveillance of the upper urinary tract is crucial and sometimes difficult endoscopically, and requires a general anesthetic. In addition, carcinoma in situ of the ureter is frequently missed when using the ureteroscope. Most tumors are high grade, however, and are treated by nephroureterectomy with the exception of distal third ureteral tumors where a distal ureterectomy and reimplantation of the ureter can be utilized. Metastatic disease is also responsive to MVAC (methotrexate, vinblastine, Adriamycin [doxorubicin], and cisplatin) chemotherapy.

BLADDER CANCER

CONSULTANTS: Bernard Lytton, M.D.—Urologist
David Esrig, M.D.—Urologist

The second most common tumor of the genitourinary tract (second only to prostate cancer); overall, the fifth most common cancer and the eleventh most common cause of cancer mortality.

Note: Incidence and new case statistics available lump together both in situ and invasive tumors because coders have not separated them in reporting.

INCIDENCE AND SURVIVAL

	Total	Male	Female
Incidence rate per 100,000/yr	16.9	29.9	7.5
Mortality rate per 100,000/yr	3.3	5.7	1.7
New cancer cases (ACS est 1994)	51,200	38,000	13,200
Cancer deaths (ACS est 1994)	10,600	7800	3600
5-year relative survival rates by stage			
All stages	78.8%	80.6%	73.7%
Localized	90.6%	91.4%	88.3%
Regional	45.9%	47.3%	42.5%
Distant	9.4%	11.9%	4.4%
Unstaged	59.9%	66.1%	47.6%

Trends

Incidence has increased very slightly and mortality has decreased greatly.

Major risk factors

Tobacco smoking accounts for about half of all cases of bladder cancer in males and one-third of those in females. Occupational exposure to aniline dyes accounts for 10% of the cases in men. Ionizing radiation, phenacetin abuse, and cyclophosphamide cause some cases. In the Middle East and Africa, especially Egypt, infection with *Schistosomiasis haematobium* is a causative factor in most cases of squamous cell carcinoma.

Pathology (major types)

Transitional cell carcinoma (90%), squamous cell carcinoma (6–8%), adenocarcinoma (2%).

Metastatic sites (major)

Regional lymph nodes, lung, liver, and bone.

Associated malignancies

Urethra, lung, pharynx, esophagus, and kidney.

Therapy

Surgery, intravesical chemotherapy or immunotherapy, systemic chemotherapy, and radiation.

Recommendations to patient

Avoid smoking. Long-term surveillance is required to detect late recurrence.

Recommendations to family

Avoid smoking.

FOLLOW-UP OF THE PATIENT WITH BLADDER CANCER

	1st Year (Months)				2nd–5th Year (Months)		Thereafter (Months)
	3	6	9	12	6	12	12
Hisotry							
Complete				×		×	×
Hematuria	×	×	×		×		
Dysuria	×	×	×		×		
Frequency	×	×	×		×		
Bone pain	×	×	×		×		
Physical							
Complete				×		×	×
Abdomen	×	×	×		×		
Rectal	×	×	×		×		
Stoma (if any)	×	×	×		×		
Lymph nodes	×	×	×		×		
Cystoscopy*	×	×		×	×	×	×
Ureteroscopy		×		×	As indicated		
Pelvic (female)		×		×	×	×	×
Tests							
Chest x-ray				×		×	×
CBC		×		×		×	×
Urine	×	×	×	×	×	×	×
BUN, alkaline phosphatase		×		×		×	×
IVP**				×		×	×
Urine cytology		×		×		×	

*This should revert to the initial follow-up, ie, every 3 months for the first 6 months after each occurrence.
**IVP should be performed at 3 months following a urinary diversion and at 6-month intervals in the first year for upper-tract tumors.

Comments: Carcinoma of the bladder is the most frequent tumor of this group and the majority are transitional cell tumors. Most cases involve only the mucosa and are treated by resection or fulguration through the cystoscope. When superficial noninvasive tumors are recurrent or multifocal, topical chemotherapy (thiotepa, mitomycin, or doxorubicin) or topical immunotherapy (BCG) may provide effective control. Careful surveillance is essential to detect invasion of the bladder wall, which requires cystectomy or radiation therapy to prevent metastatic spread. Metastatic disease is treated by combination chemotherapy (MVAC: methotrexate, vinblastine, Adriamycin [doxorubicin], and cisplatin), which has proved to be very effective. It is also being used successfully as adjuvant therapy in a variety of protocols, the long-term results of which are encouraging.

URETHRAL CANCER

CONSULTANT: Joseph D. Schmidt, M.D.—Urologist

An uncommon neoplasm and the only cancer of the urinary system that is more frequent in women than men (3:1 or 4:1).

INCIDENCE AND SURVIVAL

	Total
5-year survival rate by location	
Anterior urethra	50–66%
Posterior urethra	10–15%

Trends

The rarity of these tumors makes it difficult to gather any reliable statistics. Combination chemotherapy is now being tried for posterior tumors in hopes of improving responses and survival.

Major risk factors

Chronic irritation, obstruction, and infection; urethral stricture and urethral diverticulae.

Pathology (major types)

In the male, squamous cell carcinoma (78%), transitional cell carcinoma (15%), adenocarcinoma (6%), and undifferentiated carcinoma (1%). In the female, squamous cell carcinoma (70%), transitional cell carcinoma (18%), and adenocarcinoma (10%).

Metastatic sites (major)

Regional lymph nodes and adjacent organs.

Therapy

Surgery, radiation, and chemotherapy. Therapy often involves urinary diversion.

Recommendations to patient

If bleeding from urethra, seek early medical care.

FOLLOW-UP OF THE PATIENT WITH URETHRAL CANCER

	1st Year (Months)				2nd Year (Months)		Thereafter (Months)
	3	6	9	12	6	12	12
History							
Complete				×		×	×
Urinary symptoms	×	×	×		×		
Pain	×	×	×		×		
Genital, leg swelling	×	×	×		×		
Appetite, weight	×	×	×		×		
Physical							
Complete				×		×	×
Inguinal lymph nodes	×	×	×		×		
Operative site	×	×	×		×		
Abdomen	×	×	×		×		
Genitalia	×	×	×		×		
Extremities	×	×	×		×		
Rectal	×	×	×		×		
Stomal exam	×	×	×		×		
Tests							
Urethral (urine) cytology*	×	×	×	×	×	×	×
Chest x-ray				×		×	×
CBC, chemistry panel		×		×		×	×
Urinalysis	×	×	×	×	×	×	×
IVP/renal ultrasound**		×		×		×	×
CT scan of abdomen and pelvis				×		×	×
Cystoscopy***	×	×	×	×	×	×	×

*Actual specimen used will depend on status of urinary tract, eg, voided urine for intact tract, conduit urine or other specimen if diverted.

**Indicated if patient has had urinary diversion.

***Indicated for patients with transitional cell carcinoma.

Comments: The prognosis of urethral cancer following definitive treatment depends on the stage, location, and size of the tumor. Posterior urethral carcinomas, since they are generally of higher stage (muscle invasion with increased risk of lymphogenous and hematogenous spread), will have a worse prognosis. Also, tumors greater than 5-cm diameter have a poor prognosis. Most local recurrence and distant metastasis occur within the first 12–24 months. Patients with transitional cell carcinoma of the urethra need to be followed for similar lesions in their remaining urinary tract. Multi-drug chemotherapy (methotrexate, cisplatin, vinblastine, and doxorubicin) may be indicated for advanced transitional cell carcinoma of the urethra.

PROSTATE CANCER

CONSULTANTS: Peter T. Scardino, M.D.—Urologist
Özdal Dillioglugil, M.D.—Urologist

The most frequently diagnosed cancer in the United States today, and the third most frequent cause of cancer deaths among men (after lung and colorectal cancer).

INCIDENCE AND SURVIVAL

	Total
Incidence rate per 100,000/yr	107.7
Mortality per 100,000/yr	20.0
New cancer cases (ACS est 1995)	244,000
Cancer deaths (ACS est 1995)	40,400
5-year relative survival rates by stage	
All stages	78.0%
Localized	93.0%
Regional	83.0%
Distant	29.0%

Trends
Increasingly a disease of older age. Mean age at diagnosis is 71 but is decreasing with earlier detection. Age-specific incidence and mortality rates continue to increase. The number of new cases and deaths per year is increasing as the population ages and other causes of death decrease.

Major risk factors
Age (prostate cancer increases with age more rapidly than any other cancer), family history (two- to threefold increase), and race (ethnic groups). Possible risk factors include increased consumption of animal fat and decreased exposure to sunlight.

Pathology (major types)
Carcinomas arise primarily in the peripheral zone. More than 95% of adenocarcinomas arise in the acinar and proximal duct epithelium. Rare variants include endometrioid and mucinous (signet ring) carcinoma. Other types include adenoid cystic, small-cell undifferentiated carcinomas, and carcinoid, which do not respond well to endocrine therapy.

Metastatic sites (major)
Local extension through capsule or via ejaculatory ducts to seminal vesicles. Regional lymph node metastases are common in locally advanced cancers. Direct spread to bladder or rectum is rare and is seen in locally extensive cancers. Distant metastases to bones of the axial skeleton are most common and are usually blastic.

Associated malignancies
Lung, colon, and bladder.

Therapy
Surgery (radical prostatectomy with or without pelvic lymphadenectomy) and radiation therapy (primary or adjuvant) for localized disease (T1-3), hormonal therapy and occasional chemotherapy for metastatic disease.

Recommendations to patient
Routine annual prostate-specific antigen (PSA) testing and digital rectal examination after age 50 (age 40 for high-risk groups such as African Americans or positive family history) for screening. Avoid supplemental androgens.

Recommendations to family
Obtain early screening if disease is of the familial type (a relative diagnosed prior to age 55 or more than one first-degree relative).

FOLLOW-UP OF THE PATIENT WITH PROSTATE CANCER

	3 Weeks	6 Weeks	1st Year (Months)			2nd–5th Year (Months)		Thereafter (Months)
			4	8	12	6	12	12
History and Counseling								
Complete					✕		✕	✕
Pain (incisional, bony)	✕	✕	✕	✕		✕		
Diarrhea	✕	✕	✕	✕		✕		
Proctalgia	✕	✕	✕					
Constipation	✕	✕						
Urinary symptoms	✕	✕	✕	✕		✕		
Continence	✕*	✕	✕	✕		✕		
Potency	✕*	✕	✕	✕		✕		
Performance status	✕	✕	✕	✕		✕		
Physical								
Complete					✕		✕	✕
Wound/XRT site	✕	✕	✕					
External genitalia	✕	✕	✕	✕				
Rectal			✕	✕		✕		
Leg swelling/calf pain	✕	✕						
Tests								
PSA	✕	✕	✕	✕	✕	✕	✕	✕
Urinalysis		✕			✕		✕	✕
Renal ultrasound	✕				✕			
Flow rate		✕	✕		✕		✕	✕
Ultrasound for PVR**								
Chest x-ray**								
Bone scan**								
Bone MRI**								
IVP**								
Needle biopsy for prostate***					✕		✕	

*Counseling.
**As indicated by clinical findings and tests (PVR: postvoiding urine residue).
***One year or 2 years after radiotherapy (XRT) or whenever it is indicated after radical prostatectomy.

Comments: Serial PSA testing is indispensable in the follow-up after therapy; a fall in values indicates a favorable response; a rise indicates recurrence. After radical prostatectomy, serum PSA should become undetectable. Recurrence, whether local or distant, is preceded by a rising PSA years before any other evidence of recurrence. Local recurrence is best detected by rectal examination, but most recurrences are distant (bones or lymph nodes), especially in patients with a high-grade cancer or advanced pathologic stage. If PSA rises in the absence of clinical recurrence, a needle biopsy of the anastomotic area is done to rule out microscopic local recurrence, which can be treated with local radiotherapy. After radiotherapy, serum PSA levels should fall below the upper limit of normal within 6 months to 2 years. The PSA nadir correlates with prognosis. A rising level signals local or distant recurrence. Local recurrence is best detected by needle biopsy, which may document persistent cancer even when the PSA level is low. Local recurrence alone can be treated with salvage radical surgery or palliatively with androgen deprivation. Other tests, including bone scans, chest films, KUB, or IVP are rarely (if ever) positive in the absence of a rising PSA or clinical symptoms, and need not be done routinely. Treatment with androgen deprivation therapy is usually initiated when the PSA level rises before the local or distant recurrence can be documented. The prostatic acid phosphatase test is of little additional value.

PENILE CANCER
CONSULTANT: William R. Fair, M.D.—Urologist

This tumor is very rare in circumcised males. It represents 2–5% of all urogenital cancers in North America.

INCIDENCE AND SURVIVAL

	Total
Incidence rate per 100,000/yr	0.7
Mortality rate per 100,000/yr	0.2
New cancer cases (est 1990)	<1300
Cancer deaths (est 1990)	<200
5-year relative survival rates by stage	
All stages	70%
Localized	80%
Regional	52%
Distant	18%

Trends
This cancer is preventable and should decrease in incidence with improved hygiene, improved socioeconomic levels, and the practice of circumcision early in life.

Major risk factors
Phimosis. HIV. Premalignant lesions (Bowen's disease, Queyrat's erythroplasia, Buschke-Löwenstein's tumor), leukoplakia, and balanitis xerotica.

Pathology (major types)
Squamous cell carcinoma (90%+), transitional cell carcinoma, adenocarcinoma, Kaposi's sarcoma, and melanoma.

Metastatic sites (major)
Regional lymph nodes, especially inguinal. Lung, liver, and bone.

Therapy
Surgery, radiation, and chemotherapy.

Recommendations to patient
Avoid phimosis.

Recommendations to family
Practice early-life circumcision. (It should be noted that the practice of early-life circumcision as a medical preventive procedure is less common in the United States in recent years on the presumption that adequate hygiene will obviate the problem. The author and consultant both agree that early-life circumcision remains a worthwhile prophylactic procedure, although perhaps less compelling than it was when good hygiene was more difficult.)

FOLLOW-UP OF THE PATIENT WITH PENILE CANCER

	1st Year (Months)				2nd Year (Months)		Thereafter (Months)
	3	6	9	12	6	12	12
History							
Complete				×		×	×
Urinary symptoms	×	×	×		×		
Pain	×	×	×		×		
Leg swelling	×	×	×		×		
Appetite, weight	×	×	×		×		
Physical							
Complete				×		×	×
Lymph nodes	×	×	×		×		
Operative site	×	×	×		×		
Abdomen	×	×	×		×		
Leg edema	×	×	×		×		
Rectal	×	×	×		×		
Tests							
Chest x-ray		×		×		×	×
CBC				×		×	×
Urine	×	×	×	×	×	×	×
CT of abdomen and pelvis		×		×		×	Yearly for 4 years
Stool for blood	×	×	×	×	×	×	×

Comments: It is important to emphasize the need for monthly self-examination, especially of the inguinal area, and the penis itself, particularly in patients who had a partial penectomy. Monthly self-examinations are the cornerstone of the detection of early metastatic spread. Unlike many cancers, it is well demonstrated that metastatic spread of penile or scrotal cancer to the inguinal lymph nodes can be cured by regional lymphadenectomy. However, once the deep pelvic nodes are involved, the likelihood of cure is minimal. Since the status of the lymph nodes is so significantly related to eventual curability of the disease, it is best to do a CT scan of both the abdomen (for abdominal lymphadenopathy) and pelvic lymph nodes at 6 and 12 months the first year, and then yearly thereafter for 5 years. This makes an IVP superfluous. Although late recurrences are the exception rather than the rule, recurrences beyond 2 years are not uncommon, and even in a patient who is conscientious about inguinal self-examination, the presence of inguinal lymphadenopathy can often be seen on CT scan before it can be palpated by the patient, especially in obese patients.

Testicular Cancer

Consultant: Lawrence H. Einhorn, M.D.—Medical Oncologist

Accounts for 1% of malignancies in males and is the most frequently occurring cancer in males between the ages of 15 and 35. At one time, testicular cancer had a very limited survival rate, but with chemotherapy and a better understanding of the disease, it is now one of the most curable cancers.

INCIDENCE AND SURVIVAL

	Total
Incidence rate per 100,000/yr	4.4
Mortality rate per 100,000/yr	0.3
New cancer cases (ACS est 1994)	6800
Cancer deaths (ACS est 1994)	325
5-year relative survival rates by stage	
All stages	92.5%
Localized	97.4%
Regional	94.8%
Distant	67.4%
Unstaged	82.9%

Trends

Incidence is increasing but mortality rates are decreasing. Survival continues to improve with treatment.

Major risk factors

Cryptorchidism, atrophic testis.

Pathology (major types)

Seminoma (30%), embryonal cell carcinoma (30%), teratoma (10%), teratocarcinoma (25%), choriocarcinoma (1%); remaining 5% include Leydig cell tumors, Sertoli cell tumors, mixed tumors (variable).

Metastatic sites (major)

Regional lymph nodes, lung, liver, bone, and brain.

Associated malignancies

Extragonadal germ cell tumors.

Therapy

Surgery, chemotherapy, and radiation.

Recommendations to patient

Periodic chest x-rays, mediastinal CT scans, and tumor marker studies are essential for follow-up.

Recommendations to family

Beta-HCG levels may be elevated in persons who use marijuana.

FOLLOW-UP OF THE PATIENT WITH TESTICULAR CANCER

Following orchiectomy alone for clinical stage I disease with close surveillance, or orchiectomy followed by retroperitoneal lymph node dissection for stage I–II disease, if no adjuvant chemotherapy is given, then follow-up for these cases should be monthly history and physical examination, PA and lateral chest x-ray, and serum HCG and AFP during the first postoperative year, every 2 months the second year, every 6 months for years 3 to 5, and then annually. Since 1–2% of cured testis patients will develop a second primary in the contralateral testis, history should include discussion of the remaining testicle and physical examination should include its palpation.

When surveillance (orchiectomy alone) is employed, an abdominal CT should be done every 2 months the first year, every 4 months the second year, and every 6 months for years 3 to 5.

If adjuvant chemotherapy is given for pathological stage II, follow-up is done every 3 months the first year, every 6 months the second, and then annually.

If a complete remission is achieved with chemotherapy for metastatic testis cancer, the relapse rate is only 10%. Follow-up is done every 2 months the first year, every 4 months the second year, every 6 months for years 3 to 5, and then annually. There is no need to repeat abdominal CT scans following a complete remission after chemotherapy.

Comments: Since early-stage testicular seminomas are cured in 90–95% of patients by orchiectomy with chemotherapy or radiation, and 90% of nonseminomatous germ cell tumors (NSGCT) are curable by orchiectomy and retroperitoneal lymphadenectomy (RPLND) or chemotherapy, or a combination of both, meticulous follow-up with chest x-rays and tumor markers is essential for at least the first 2 years, and probably for an additional 3 years. This is particularly important in patients who opt for surveillance after orchiectomy rather than RPLND. Patients with recurrent disease, including small distant metastases, have been rendered disease-free by aggressive combination chemotherapy and have enjoyed prolonged survival. If a patient who has completed therapy remains free of disease for 3 years after treatment, his probability of cure is greater than 95%.

For an alternative follow-up program, see the discussion of extragonadal and gonadal germ cell tumors beginning on the next page.

EXTRAGONADAL AND GONADAL GERM CELL TUMORS

CONSULTANT: George J. Bosl, M.D.—Medical Oncologist

Testicular germ cell tumors are the most common tumors in men between the ages of 15 and 35. Extragonadal germ cell tumors can arise in the retroperitoneum, mediastinum, pineal gland, stomach, prostate, and thymus. They are often difficult to find clinically and sometimes hard to identify histologically. They represent 3% of malignant diseases in childhood and adolescence. Pathologically they are identical to testicular germ cell tumors. With modern chemotherapy, careful attention to follow-up, and appropriately timed surgical intervention, more than 90% of all newly diagnosed germ cell tumor patients will be cured of disease. Above the age of 50 years old, a testicular mass is a lymphoma until proven otherwise. Cryptorchidism is the only proven risk factor, although an atrophic testis and a family history may place a patient at higher risk. Ninety-five percent of testicular tumors are germ cell tumors and the remaining 5% include stromal tumors and others. Pure seminomas account for about 40% of the germ cell tumors while single and mixed nonseminomatous cell types account for the remainder. Alpha-fetoprotein (AFP) and human chorionic gonadotropin (HCG) and its beta subunit (beta-HCG) are highly specific tumor markers for patients with nonseminomatous germ cell tumors; AFP is never produced by pure seminomas whereas HCG may be produced by an occasional seminoma. Lactic dehydrogenase (LDH) is also a useful, but somewhat less specific, tumor marker. It is elevated with equal frequency in seminomas and nonseminomas, and it is an important prognostic variable. The primary nodal drainage is to the retroperitoneum. Subsequent metastatic sites include the supraclavicular lymph nodes, lung, and other visceral sites.

Pathology (major types)

Seminoma, embryonal cell carcinoma, teratoma, choriocarcinoma, endodermal sinus tumor (yolk sac tumor), nonseminomatous germ cell tumors are usually composed of several histologic types (mixed germ cell tumors).

Metastatic sites (major)

Lung, mediastinum, retroperitoneum, bone, supralavicular nodes, and brain.

Associated malignancies

Malignant hematologic dyscrasias may arise from a mediastinal nonseminomatous germ cell tumor. Sarcomas and carcinomas of various histologic types may arise from mature teratoma (malignant transformation).

Therapy

Chemotherapy, surgery, and radiation.

Recommendations to patient

Do not smoke, especially if bleomycin was included in chemotherapy regimen.

FOLLOW-UP OF THE PATIENT WITH SEMINOMA RECEIVING RADIATION THERAPY

	1st Year (Months)						2nd Year (Months)				3rd Year (Months)		4th Year (and annually)
	0	2	4	6	9	12	3	6	9	12	6	12	12
History													
Back pain	×	×	×	×	×	×	×	×	×	×	×	×	×
Nipple tenderness	×	×	×	×	×	×	×	×	×	×	×	×	×
Cough	×	×	×	×	×	×	×	×	×	×	×	×	×
Abdominal pain	×	×	×	×	×	×	×	×	×	×	×	×	×
Physical													
Nodes	×	×	×	×	×	×	×	×	×	×	×	×	×
Lungs	×	×	×	×	×	×	×	×	×	×	×	×	×
Breasts	×	×	×	×	×	×	×	×	×	×	×	×	×
Abdomen	×	×	×	×	×	×	×	×	×	×	×	×	×
Testes*	×	×	×	×	×	×	×	×	×	×	×	×	×
Tests													
CBC (if prior chemo/RT)	×	×	×	×	×	×	×	×	×	×	×	×	×
Chest x-ray	×	×	×	×	×	×	×	×	×	×	×	×	×
Beta-HCG	×	×	×	×	×	×	×	×	×	×	×	×	×
Alpha-fetoprotein	×	×	×	×	×	×	×	×	×	×	×	×	×
LDH	×	×	×	×	×	×	×	×	×	×	×	×	×
CT of abdomen**	×	×											

*Two percent of all patients develop a second primary tumor. Self-exam should be taught to all patients.
**Not generally needed in patients with prior retroperitoneal lymph node dissection or RT.

Comments: Follow-up is an extremely important part of the management of patients with germ cell tumors. Given the curability of this disease with initial therapy and the availability of curative second-line and even third-line (bone marrow transplant) therapy, attention to detail in follow-up is important in order to detect minimal recurrent disease.

Follow-up procedures are the same for germ cell tumors of both extragonadal and gonadal origin. Extragonadal seminoma has the same prognosis as testicular seminoma; extragonadal nonseminomas denote a poor risk status and require more intensive therapy. Nonetheless, patients who achieve complete remission after radiation therapy or chemotherapy may be monitored with similar follow-up strategies regardless of the site of origin or the treatment that is used.

FOLLOW-UP OF THE PATIENT WITH NONSEMINOMATOUS GERM CELL TUMORS AND SEMINOMAS REQUIRING CHEMOTHERAPY

	1st Year (Months)											
	0	1	2	3	4	5	6	[7]	8	[9]	10	[11]	12
History													
Back pain	×	×	×	×	×	×	×	[×]	×	[×]	×	[×]	×
Nipple tenderness	×	×	×	×	×	×	×	[×]	×	[×]	×	[×]	×
Cough	×	×	×	×	×	×	×	[×]	×	[×]	×	[×]	×
Abdominal pain	×	×	×	×	×	×	×	[×]	×	[×]	×	[×]	×
Physical													
Nodes	×	×	×	×	×	×	×	[×]	×	[×]	×	[×]	×
Lungs	×	×	×	×	×	×	×	[×]	×	[×]	×	[×]	×
Breasts	×	×	×	×	×	×	×	[×]	×	[×]	×	[×]	×
Abdomen	×	×	×	×	×	×	×	[×]	×	[×]	×	[×]	×
Testes*	×	×	×	×	×	×	×	[×]	×	[×]	×	[×]	×
Tests													
CBC**	×	×	×	×	×	×	×	[×]	×	[×]	×	[×]	×
Chest x-ray	×	×	×	×	×	×	×	[×]	×	[×]	×	[×]	×
Beta-HCG	×	×	×	×	×	×	×	[×]	×	[×]	×	[×]	×
Alpha-fetoprotein	×	×	×	×	×	×	×	[×]	×	[×]	×	[×]	×
LDH	×	×	×	×	×	×	×	[×]	×	[×]	×	[×]	×
CT of abdomen***	×			[×]			[×]			[×]			[×]

*Two percent of all patients develop a second primary tumor. Self-exam should be taught to all patients.
**CBC if prior chemotherapy or radiation therapy.
***Needed only in patients who are being observed with clinical stage I nonseminomatous germ cell tumors.
[ ]Not needed in patients treated with adjuvant chemotherappy for pathologic nonseminomatous stage II B disease.

2nd Year (Months)						3rd Year (Months)				4th Year (Months)		5th Year (and annually)
[2]	4	[6]	8	[10]	12	[3]	6	[9]	12	[6]	12	12
[×]	×	[×]	×	[×]	×	[×]	×	[×]	×	[×]	×	×
[×]	×	[×]	×	[×]	×	[×]	×	[×]	×	[×]	×	×
[×]	×	[×]	×	[×]	×	[×]	×	[×]	×	[×]	×	×
[×]	×	[×]	×	[×]	×	[×]	×	[×]	×	[×]	×	×
[×]	×	[×]	×	[×]	×	[×]	×	[×]	×	[×]	×	×
[×]	×	[×]	×	[×]	×	[×]	×	[×]	×	[×]	×	×
[×]	×	[×]	×	[×]	×	[×]	×	[×]	×	[×]	×	×
[×]	×	[×]	×	[×]	×	[×]	×	[×]	×	[×]	×	×
[×]	×	[×]	×	[×]	×	[×]	×	[×]	×	[×]	×	×
[×]	×	[×]	×	[×]	×	[×]	×	[×]	×	[×]	×	×
[×]	×	[×]	×	[×]	×	[×]	×	[×]	×	[×]	×	×
[×]	×	[×]	×	[×]	×	[×]	×	[×]	×	[×]	×	×
[×]	×	[×]	×	[×]	×	[×]	×	[×]	×	[×]	×	×
[×]	×	[×]	×	[×]	×	[×]	×	[×]	×	[×]	×	×
	[×]		[×]		[×]		[×]		[×]	[×]	[×]	[×]

7

GYNECOLOGIC CANCERS

OVARIAN EPITHELIAL CANCER

Consultant: Peter E. Schwartz, M.D.—Gynecological Oncologist

The fourth most common cause of cancer death in women and the leading cause of all female genital cancer deaths in the United States. One in 70 women will develop ovarian cancer in her lifetime.

INCIDENCE AND SURVIVAL

	Total		
Incidence rate per 100,000/yr	14.3		
Mortality rate per 100,000/yr	7.8		
New cancer cases (ACS est 1994)	24,000		
Cancer deaths (ACS est 1994)	13,600		
		Under Age 50	**Above Age 50**
5-year relative survival rates by stage			
All stages	39.2%	64.2%	31.5%
Localized	88.4%	91.3%	86.7%
Regional	36.4%	60.5%	30.7%
Distant	17.4%	35.4%	13.5%
Unstaged	21.7%	54.9%	15.1%

Trends

Decreased mortality and increased survival over the past two decades with no change in incidence suggests slight increases in cure rates, primarily in younger women.

Major risk factors

Familial predisposition, infertility, nulliparity, older age, early age of menarche, late age of menopause, Western European or North American descent.

Pathology (major types)

Epithelial carcinomas of the ovary account for 80–90% of ovarian malignancies while germ cell (4–7%) and stromal cell cancers account for the remainder. Epithelial cancers of serous, mucinous, endometrioid, or clear cell type may be aggressive adenocarcinomas or tumors of low malignancy.

Metastatic sites (major)

Contiguous and transperitoneal organs, pelvic and para-aortic lymph nodes, diaphragm, lung, liver, serosa, pleura, peritoneum overlying the kidneys, adrenal glands, bladder, and spleen.

Associated malignancies

Breast, endometrial, and colon.

Therapy

Surgery, radiation, and chemotherapy.

Recommendations to patient

Avoid obesity.

Recommendations to family

Seek genetic counseling to evaluate risk and clarify options for prevention. Consider birth control pills for contraception at an early age and tubal ligation for permanent sterilization.

FOLLOW-UP OF THE PATIENT WITH OVARIAN EPITHELIAL CANCER

	1st Year (Months)				2nd–5th Year (Months)		Thereafter (Months)	
	3	6	9	12	6	12	6	12
History								
Complete				×	×		×	
Increase abdominal size/masses	×	×	×		×			
Pelvic pain	×	×	×		×			
Vaginal bleeding	×	×	×		×			
Weight gain or loss	×	×	×		×			
Leg edema	×	×	×		×			
Changes in appetite	×	×	×		×			
Physical								
Complete				×	×		×	
Pelvic exam	×	×	×		×			
Abdomen	×	×	×		×			
Lymph nodes	×	×	×		×			
Breasts	×	×	×		×			
Extremities	×	×	×		×			
Tests								
Chest x-ray				×	×			×
CT scan abdomen*	As indicated							
CBC		×		×	×	×	×	×
CA-125	×	×	×	×	×	×	×	×
Pap smear	Every two years							

*As indicated unless original tumor did not express CA-125.

Comments: The primary goal of follow-up is the early detection of recurrent tumor, hopefully at a time when further treatment offers the possibility of disease control. To this end, the patient must be made an active partner in follow-up, impressed with the responsibility to report promptly any new or persistent symptom for the physician's evaluation. Lifelong follow-up on a regular programmed schedule is important. The majority of advanced-stage ovarian carcinoma patients will develop recurrent disease within 2 years. Rising CA-125 levels are highly suggestive of recurrent disease. For most ovarian cancers treated with adjuvant chemotherapy, a normal physical exam, CT scan, and CA-125 titers may obviate the need for second-look laparotomy.

OVARIAN LOW MALIGNANT POTENTIAL TUMOR

CONSULTANT: William J. Hoskins, M.D.—Gynecological Oncologist

Accounts for 15–20% of all epithelial ovarian carcinomas. About 75% are stage I at time of diagnosis.

SURVIVAL	Total
Mortality rate per 100,000/year	
Stage I	0.7%
Stage II	4.2%
Stage III	26.8%
Survival rate	
At 5 years	97%
At 10 years	95%
At 15 years	92%
At 20 years	89%
5-year relative survival rates by stage	
Stage I	95–98%
Stages II–IV (grouped)	65%

Trends

Increasing incidence may be due to improved diagnosis and recognition.

Major risk factors

Familial predisposition, infertility, and nulliparity.

Pathology (major types)

Serous, mucinous, and endometrioid.

Metastatic sites (major)

Rarely, nodes, diaphragm, lung, liver, bone, pleura, mediastinal lymph nodes, peritoneum overlying kidneys, adrenal glands, bladder, and spleen.

Associated malignancies

Breast, endometrial, and colon cancer.

Therapy

Surgery, radiation, and chemotherapy.

Recommendations to patients

Avoid obesity.

Recommendations to family

Seek genetic counseling to evaluate risk and clarify options for prevention.

FOLLOW-UP OF THE PATIENT WITH OVARIAN LOW MALIGNANT POTENTIAL TUMORS

	1st Year (Months)		2nd–5th Year (Months)		Thereafter (Months)
	6	12	6	12	12
History					
Complete		×		×	×
Increase abdominal size/masses	×		×		
Pelvic pain	×		×		
Vaginal bleeding	×		×		
Weight gain or loss	×		×		
Leg edema	×		×		
Changes in appetite	×		×		
Physical					
Complete		×		×	×
Pelvic exam	×		×		
Abdomen	×		×		
Lymph nodes	×		×		
Breast	×		×		
Extremities	×		×		
Tests					
Chest x-ray		×		×	×
CT scan of abdomen	Only indicated for stage III and IV disease				
CBC	Only if chemotherapy was given				
Pap smear		×		×	×
CA-125	×	×	×	×	×

Comments: Ovarian tumors of low malignant potential have a very slow growth rate and recur rarely and late. Patients with stage I disease almost never recur. Even patients with advanced disease (stages III and IV) usually recur quite late (3–6 years).

OVARIAN GERM CELL CANCER

CONSULTANT: David M. Gershenson, M.D.—Gynecological Oncologist

Accounts for about 5% of all ovarian malignancies in the United States. Incidence is much higher in the Orient, where up to 15% of ovarian cancers are of the germ cell type.

SURVIVAL

	Total
Overall survival rate	85% at 5 years
5-year relative survival rates by stage	
Stage I	95+%
Stage II	95+%
Stage III	75–80%
Stage IV	60%

Major risk factors

Occurs in younger women. Most of the ovarian cancers that occur in women age 30 or younger are germ cell cancers. Gonadal dysgenesis and androgen insensitivity syndrome predispose to dysgerminoma or other germ cell tumors.

Pathology (major types)

Dysgerminoma, endodermal sinus tumor, immature teratoma, mixed germ cell tumors, embryonal carcinoma, nongestational choriocarcinoma, and polyembryoma.

Metastatic sites (major)

Retroperitoneal nodes, peritoneal surfaces; less frequently, lung, mediastinal and supraclavicular lymph nodes, bone, brain, and liver.

Associated malignancies

Slightly increased risk of acute nonlymphocytic and acute myelomonocytic leukemia related to chemotherapy.

Therapy

Surgery and chemotherapy.

Recommendations to patient

Follow-up with tumor markers, alpha-fetoprotein, and/or beta-HCG is advisable early to detect persistent or recurrent germ cell tumors if initially elevated.

Recommendations to family

Currently, there is no known genetic or familial aspect associated with this category of tumors.

FOLLOW-UP OF THE PATIENT WITH OVARIAN GERM CELL CANCER

	First 2 Years (Months)												3rd–5th Year (Months)			Thereafter (Months)
	1	2	3	4	5	6	7	8	9	10	11	12	4	8	12	12
History																
Complete												X		X		X
Abdominal pain	X	X	X	X	X	X	X	X	X	X	X		X	X		
Abdominal size	X	X	X	X	X	X	X	X	X	X	X	X	X	X		
Vaginal bleeding	X	X	X	X	X	X	X	X	X	X	X		X	X		
Physical																
Complete												X		X		X
Pelvic exam	X	X	X	X	X	X	X	X	X	X	X	X				
Abdomen	X	X	X	X	X	X	X	X	X	X	X	X				
Lymph nodes	X	X	X	X	X	X	X	X	X	X	X	X				
Breast												X		X		X
Tests																
Chest x-ray												X		X		X
CBC						X						X		X		X
SMA12						X						X		X		
HCG*	X	X	X	X	X	X	X	X	X	X	X	X	X	X	X	
AFP*	X	X	X	X	X	X	X	X	X	X	X	X				
Pap smear												X		X		X

*If initially elevated.

Comment: For malignant embryonal carcinoma, endodermal sinus tumors, and malignant teratomas, survival rates with surgery alone, or even with radical surgery followed by radiation therapy, are disappointing. When the tumor is confined to one ovary, unilateral salpingo-oophorectomy is the surgery of choice for the young patient. For germ cell tumors that have spread to the fallopian tube or uterus, but not to the other ovary, complete tumor removal without total hysterectomy or removal of the uninvolved adnexae is indicated. These patients can usually be cured with combination chemotherapy with preservation of their reproductive function.

Early stage dysgerminomas may be curable by surgery alone. Although sensitive to radiation therapy, more advanced dysgerminomas are generally treated with combination chemotherapy succesfully and often with preservation of reproductive function. Failures or recurrences are treated with radiation therapy alone or in combination with a non-cross reactive chemotherapy program.

All patients with germ cell tumors should be followed carefully because therapy for recurrence is frequently highly effective in prolongation of survival.

ENDOMETRIAL CANCER
CONSULTANT: William T. Creasman, M.D.—Gynecological Oncologist

The most common malignancy of the female genital system, representing 46% of all female genital cancers and 11% of all malignancies in women, but only 23% of gynecologic cancer deaths.

INCIDENCE AND SURVIVAL

	Total	
Incidence rate per 100,000/yr	21.2	
Mortality rate per 100,000/yr	3.3	
New cancer cases (ACS est 1994)	31,000	
Cancer deaths (ACS est 1994)	5900	
Survival rates by stage	3 Years (%)	5 Years (%)
Stage I	83.2	76.3
Stage II	69.0	59.2
Stage III	37.1	29.4
Stage IV	14.2	10.3
Unstaged	60.1	51.8

Trends
Both incidence and mortality have decreased over the past two decades.

Major risk factors
Unopposed estrogen, tamoxifen, high socioeconomic status, older age, nulliparity, infertility, menstrual irregularities, early age of menarche, late age of menopause, obesity, Stein-Leventhal syndrome (polycystic ovary disease), and functional ovarian tumors (granulosa cell tumors and thecomas).

Pathology (major types)
Endometrioid adenocarcinoma (75%), adenosquamous carcinoma (18%), clear cell carcinoma (1%), papillary serous carcinoma (6%).

Metastatic sites (major)
Adnexae, ovaries, pelvic and paraaortic nodes, peritoneum, lung, liver, and bone.

Associated malignancies
Breast, ovary, and colon.

Therapy
Surgery, radiation, chemotherapy, and hormonal therapy.

Recommendations to patient
Avoid obesity.

FOLLOW-UP OF THE PATIENT WITH ENDOMETRIAL CANCER

	1st Year (Months)				2nd Year (Months)			3rd Year (Months)		Thereafter (Months)
	3	6	9	12	4	8	12	6	12	12
History										
Complete				×			×		×	×
Vaginal bleeding	×	×	×		×	×		×		
Pelvic pain	×	×	×		×	×		×		
Abdominal size	×	×	×		×	×		×		
Hormonal medication	×	×	×		×	×		×		
Leg edema	×	×	×		×	×		×		
Physical										
Complete				×			×		×	×
Pelvic exam	×	×	×		×	×		×		
Abdomen	×	×	×		×	×		×		
Lymph nodes	×	×	×		×	×		×		
Breasts	×	×	×		×	×		×		
Rectal	×	×	×		×	×		×		
Tests										
Stool for blood	×	×	×	×	×	×	×	×	×	×
Pap smear	×	×	×	×	×	×	×	×	×	×
CA-125	As indicated									

Comments: Although a Pap smear may show malignant cells in a patient with endometrial carcinoma, it is not a sensitive test for this tumor, but rather for cervical carcinoma. Unexplained vaginal bleeding, especially in the postmenopausal patient, should be evaluated by a gynecologist and probably should include endometrial aspiration cytology or dilatation and curettage. Most recurrences are within 3 years, but may appear 10 years after initial diagnosis. Vaginal recurrence is often associated with distant disease. Unfortunately, most common recurrences are at a distant site. Today, most would not do routine chest x-ray, CBC, or urine during follow-up unless indicated. CA-125 is not done unless indicated. For those at low risk for recurrence, it is not cost-effective.

UTERINE SARCOMA

CONSULTANT: Gregory P. Sutton, M.D.—Gynecological Oncologist

Accounts for less than 1% of all gynecologic malignances and 2–5% of all uterine malignancies.

SURVIVAL

	Total
5-year overall survival rate	About 37%
5-year relative survival rates by stage	
Stage I	50%
Stage II	0–20%
Stage III	0–10%
Stage IV	0–5%

Major risk factors

Prior radiation therapy (applies to mixed müllerian tumors only).

Pathology (major types)

Mixed müllerian tumor (50%), leiomyosarcoma (30%), endometrial stromal sarcomas (15%).

Metastatic sites (major)

Adjacent organs, lung, and abdomen.

Therapy

Somewhat different for each type.

Mixed müllerian tumors: total abdominal hysterectomy (TAH) and bilateral salpingo-oophorectomy (BSO) with lymphadenectomy (nodes) and postoperative radiation therapy (RT). Stages I and II: pelvic RT. Stages III and IV: small residual—whole-abdomen RT or chemotherapy (chemoRx) with ifosfamide and cisplatin; large residual—chemoRX with ifosfamide and cisplatin. Recurrent disease: chemoRx with ifosfamide and cisplatin.

Leiomyosarcoma: TAH and BSO with or without nodes; chest x-ray; no beneficial adjuvant therapy. Recurrent disease: chemoRx with doxorubicin and ifosfamide.

Endometrial stromal sarcoma: low grade—TAH and BSO with nodes and progestogen (megestrol) with or without RT; high grade—TAH and BSO with nodes and RT. Stages I and II: pelvic RT. Stages III and IV: small volume—whole abdomen RT; large volume—chemoRx with doxorubicin and ifosfamide.

Recommendations to patient

Have gynecological examinations at periodic intervals based on age and risk. Women who have had a hysterectomy for benign disease should have a Pap smear every 3 years.

FOLLOW-UP OF THE PATIENT WITH UTERINE SARCOMA

	1st Year (Months)				2nd Year (Months)			3rd–5th Year (Months)		Thereafter (Months)
	3	6	9	12	4	8	12	6	12	12
History										
Complete				X			X		X	X
Vaginal bleeding	X	X	X		X	X		X		
Pelvic pain	X	X	X		X	X		X		
Abdominal size	X	X	X		X	X		X		
Hormonal medication	X	X	X		X	X		X		
Leg edema	X	X	X		X	X		X		
GI and GU symptoms	X	X	X		X	X		X		
Physical										
Complete				X			X		X	X
Pelvic pain	X	X	X		X	X		X		
Abdomen	X	X	X		X	X		X		
Lymph nodes	X	X	X		X	X		X		
Breasts	X	X	X		X	X		X		
Tests										
Chest x-ray				X			X		X	X
Stool for blood	X	X		X	X	X	X	X	X	X
Pap smear	X	X	X	X	X	X	X	X	X	X
CA-125	X	X	X	X	X	X	X	X	X	X
Urine	X	X		X			X		X	X

Comments: Although a Pap smear may show malignant cells in a patient with uterine sarcoma, it is not a sensitive test for this tumor, but rather for cervical carcinoma. Unexplained vaginal bleeding, especially in the postmenopausal patient, should be evaluated by a gynecologist, including endometrial biopsy or cervical colposcopy. Most recurrences are within 2 years, but may appear 10 years after initial diagnosis.

Vaginal recurrence is often associated with distant disease. The most common site of recurrence for mixed müllerian tumors (MMT) is the pelvis or vaginal apex. The most common site of recurrence of uterine leiomyosarcomas is the lung. Recurrences are usually fatal, but palliative chemotherapy with cisplatin/ifosfamide in MMT and doxorubicin/ifosfamide in leiomyosarcoma may be beneficial. Palliative radiation therapy is also used occasionally. Diagnosis, treatment, and follow-up of these patients should be done by a gynecologic oncologist.

GESTATIONAL TROPHOBLASTIC TUMOR

CONSULTANTS: Donald P. Goldstein, M.D.—Gynecological Oncologist
Ross S. Berkowitz, M.D.—Gynecological Oncologist

Hydatidiform mole (molar pregnancy [MP]), invasive mole (IM), choriocarcinoma (CCA), and placental site trophoblastic tumor (PSTT) constitute a unique group of biologically and morphologically interrelated conditions known as gestational trophoblastic tumors (GTTs). They all make human chorionic gonadotropin (HCG), which is a reliable marker for diagnosis, monitoring therapy, and follow-up. GTTs, either CCA or PSTT, develop after miscarriages (1 per 5000 pregnancies), ectopic pregnancies (1 per 15,000 pregnancies), and term gestations (1 per 150,000 live births). Morphologically, CCA consists of both cyto- and syncytial trophoblasts, while PSTT is a tumor of the intermediate trophoblast.

SURVIVAL

	Total
5-year relative survival rates by stage	
Nonmetastatic	100%
Metastatic, good prognosis	97%
Metastatic, poor prognosis	75%

Trends
Dramatically improved survival with aggressive chemotherapy and the availability of the very sensitive beta-HCG test to detect residual disease and guide therapy.

Major risk factors
Incidence increases with age, especially over age 40. Molar pregnancy, spontaneous abortion, and occasionally even a normal pregnancy. An association with inadequate carotene (vitamin A precursor) intake has been reported with MP.

Pathology (major types)
Hydatidiform mole, invasive mole, and choriocarcinoma.

Metastatic sites (major)
Lungs (80%), vagina (30%), pelvis (20%), liver (10%), brain (10%), bowel, kidney, and spleen (5%).

Therapy
Surgery, chemotherapy, and radiation therapy.

Recommendations to patient
Have abnormal vaginal bleeding checked promptly if the uterus has been retained and have gynecological examinations at periodic intervals based on age and risk status.

FOLLOW-UP OF THE PATIENT WITH GESTATIONAL TROPHOBLASTIC TUMOR

FOLLOW-UP PROCEDURE SUGGESTED

Following Molar Evacuation

Serum beta-HCG tests every week with normal results for 3 weeks, then every month for 6 months.

Following Treatment for GTT Stages I–III

1st year	Serum beta-HCG tests every month
2nd–5th year	Serum beta-HCG tests every 6 months
After 5 years	Serum beta-HCG tests every 12 months

Following Treatment for GTT Stage IV

1st–2nd year	Serum beta-HCG tests every month
3rd–4th year	Serum beta-HCG tests every 6 months
After 5 years	Serum beta-HCG tests every 12 months

Optional: Follow-up radiographic studies of lungs, liver, and brain if these organs were involved.

Comments: Metastatic disease occurs more frequently in patients who develop CCA after term pregnancy, miscarriage, and ectopics. Most often metastases are found in the lungs, vagina, pelvic cavity, GI tract, CNS, and liver. When the GI tract, brain, or liver are involved, patients are placed in the stage IV category. CNS and liver metastases are associated with poor prognosis and are treated aggressively with multimodal therapy including combination chemotherapy, surgery, and radiation therapy where indicated.

Patients with persistent disease are followed with weekly HCG values until undetectable for 3 weeks. Patients with stage I–III disease are then followed with monthly HCG levels until undetectable for 12 months. Patients with stage IV disease are monitored with monthly HCG values until undetectable for 24 months because of their greater risk for late relapse. All patients with persistent disease then continue with HCG follow-up at 6-month intervals until 5 years and then annually for life.

All other studies are optional. Certainly patients should be advised to have abnormal bleeding investigated promptly. Other signs of possible late metastases include cough, dyspnea, hemoptysis, headache or seizure activity, GI bleeding, or abdominal pain. A physical examination including a pelvic examination should be carried out at 3 months, 6 months, and 1 year, and then twice yearly for 5 years, and subsequently annually. Periodic chest x-rays may be performed if the patient had a history of lung metastases. However, in general, the absence of HCG using a sensitive and specific assay is an excellent indicator of continued sustained remission. Most relapses occur during the first year. However, there are infrequent cases in which patients develop late recurrence up to 10–15 years after treatment. Hence, lifelong annual follow-up is advised.

CERVICAL CANCER

CONSULTANTS: M. Steven Piver, M.D.—Gynecological Oncologist
Jeffrey M. Goldberg, M.D.—Gynecological Oncologist

Worldwide, cervical cancer is the most common malignancy in women. However, in the United States it accounts for only 6% of all malignancies in women and is the third most common gynecologic malignancy.

INCIDENCE AND SURVIVAL

	Total
Incidence rate per 100,000/yr	8.7
Mortality rate per 100,000/yr	3.0
New cancer cases (ACS est 1994)	15,000
Cancer deaths (ACS est 1994)	4600
5-year relative survival rates by stage	
Stage I (confined to cervix)	85%
Stage II (spread to upper vagina or paracervical tissues)	70%
Stage III (spread to lower vagina or pelvic sidewall)	50%
Stage IV (spread to bladder, rectum, or distant metastases)	<10%

Trends

Both incidence and mortality have dramatically decreased in the United States over the past several decades due to widespread use of screening with Pap smears and improvements in treatment.

Major risk factors

Multiple sexual partners, history of sexually transmitted disease (especially HPV-16, 18, and 31), early age at first intercourse, smoking, nonwhite race, low socioeconomic status.

Pathology (major types)

Squamous cell follows a relatively slowly progressive course and accounts for 90% of all tumors, but adenocarcinoma is increasing in incidence and is much more aggressive. Numerous other histologic subtypes are rare (<1–2%), but most are very aggressive with a poor prognosis.

Metastatic sites (major)

Pelvic, para-aortic, supraclavicular, then remote lymph nodes; direct extension to pelvic structures such as vagina, rectum, bladder, and ureter; lung, liver, bone, and vulva.

Associated malignancies

Vaginal cancer and vulvar cancer.

Therapy

Small stage I tumors may be treated by either radiation or radical hysterectomy. All stages are treated by radiation. Survival is improved by treatment at a major referral center with extensive experience in the treatment of cervical cancer. Chemotherapy is used only for palliation or for neoadjuvant therapy in experimental protocols.

Recommendations for patients

ACS guidelines call for annual Pap tests for 3 years beginning at age 18 or at age of first intercourse, whichever is sooner. Thereafter, Pap smears may be performed every 1–3 years at the discretion of the physician and patient. However, patients with a history of abnormal Pap smear, poor compliance with follow-up, risk factors for cervical cancer as listed above, or a partner with the same risk factors should have annual Pap smears. Abnormal Pap smears should be managed by a gynecologist with extensive experience in colposcopy and treatment of dysplasia. Invasive cancer must be managed by a gynecologic oncologist.

FOLLOW-UP OF THE PATIENT WITH CERVICAL CANCER

	1st –2nd Year (Months)				3rd–5th Year (Months)		Thereafter (Months)
	3	6	9	12	6	12	12
History							
Complete				×		×	×
Vaginal bleeding	×	×	×		×		
Bone pain	×	×	×		×		
Leg edema	×	×	×		×		
Vaginal discharge	×	×	×		×		
Appetite, weight	×	×	×		×		
Bowel function	×	×	×		×		
Bladder function	×	×	×		×		
Physical							
Complete				×		×	×
Lymph nodes	×	×	×		×		
Pelvic exam	×	×	×		×		
Abdomen	×	×	×		×		
Breasts	×	×	×		×		
Chest	×	×	×		×		
Tests							
Chest x-ray				×		×	×
CBC, chem panel		×		×	×	×	×
Pap smear	×	×	×	×	×	×	×
Urine	×	×	×	×	×	×	×
Stool for blood	×	×	×	×	×	×	×

Comments: Eighty percent of all recurrences are within 2 years of therapy. Early-stage disease is more likely to recur at distant sites rather than locally, but more advanced disease is more likely to recur locally, with or without distant metastases. Early diagnosis of local pelvic recurrence may permit successful salvage therapy. However, the only treatment for distant metastases is palliative chemotherapy or localized palliative radiation. Some authorities recommend routine screening with an IVP. However, the utility of this is unproven. In patients who develop a hydronephrosis posttreatment, approximately 70% will have hydronephrosis secondary to tumor and 30% will have hydronephrosis secondary to adhesions. Patients treated with radiation therapy should be encouraged to stay sexually active or use a dilator to keep the vagina from becoming stenotic and to permit adequate examination.

VAGINAL CANCER

CONSULTANT: Carmel J. Cohen, M.D.—Gynecological Oncologist

Accounts for 1–2% of all gynecologic malignancies.

INCIDENCE AND SURVIVAL

	Total
Incidence rate per 100,000/yr	0.6
Mortality rate per 100,00/yr	0.2
New cancer cases (est 1990)	750
Cancer deaths (est 1990)	250
5-year relative survival rates by stage	
Stage 0	100%
Stage I	94%
Stage II	80%
Stage III	50%
Stage IV A	18%
Stage IV B	10%

Trends

There is an increasing incidence of vaginal neoplasia in younger women.

Major risk factors

Vaginal adenosis from diethylstilbestrol (DES) therapy in utero, low socioeconomic status, human papillomavirus infection, prior radiation therapy.

Pathology (major types)

Squamous cell carcinoma, melanoma, clear cell carcinoma, sarcoma, lymphoma.

Metastatic sites (major)

Pelvic, inguinal, para-aortic, and supraclavicular lymph nodes, paravaginal and parametric tissues, liver, and lung.

Associated malignancies

Cervical, vulvar, bladder, and urethral cancers.

Therapy

Surgery, radiation, chemotherapy, and laser therapy.

Recommendations to patient

Have gynecological examinations at periodic intervals based on age and risk. Even women posthysterectomy for benign diseases should have a Pap smear every 3 years.

FOLLOW-UP OF THE PATIENT WITH VAGINAL CANCER

	1st Year (Months)				2nd–5th Year (Months)		Thereafter (Months)
	3	6	9	12	6	12	12
History							
Complete				×		×	×
Vaginal discharge	×	×	×		×		
Bone or pelvic pain	×	×	×		×		
Vaginal bleeding	×	×	×		×		
Appetite, weight	×	×	×		×		
Leg edema	×	×	×		×		
Bladder and bowel function	×	×	×		×		
Physical							
Complete				×		×	×
Pelvic exam	×	×	×		×		
Abdomen	×	×	×		×		
Lymph nodes	×	×	×		×		
Breasts	×	×	×		×		
Extremities	×	×	×		×		
Tests							
Chest x-ray				×		×	×
CT scan of abdomen	As indicated						
CBC		×		×	×	×	×
Pap smear		×	×	×	×	×	×

Comments: The decrease in mortality from this tumor may be attributed to better hygiene and earlier detection from routine examinations. To this end, the patient must be an active partner in the follow-up. She must be impressed with the need to return for examinations and to report promptly any new or persistent symptoms for the physician's evaluation. One-half of all recurrences may be expected within 3 years after definitive treatment, but many are seen at 5 years and some as late as 8 or 10 years or more after therapy. Thus, lifelong follow-up on a regular programmed schedule is important. Patients who were exposed to DES in utero require cytologic surveillance after initial colposcopic evaluation and selected biopsies of abnormal epithelium. Biopsy of palpable abnormalities or cytologically atypical areas should be performed during lifelong follow-up.

VULVAR CANCER

CONSULTANT: Howard D. Homesley, M.D.—Gynecological Oncologist

Accounts for 3–5% of all gynecologic malignancies and 1–2% of all malignancies in women.

INCIDENCE AND SURVIVAL

Incidence rate increases with age from 2.5 new cases per year per 100,000 of population
from ages 35–75 to 14.3 new cases per year per 100,000 of population at age 85.

	Total
Mortality rate per 100,00/yr	0.3
New cancer cases (est 1990)	2,000
Cancer deaths (est 1990)	500
5-year relative survival rates by stage	
Stage I	95%
Stage II	75–85%
Stage III	55%
Stage IV A	20%
Stage IV B	5%

Trends

Both incidence and mortality have changed little over the past two decades.

Major risk factors

Human papillomavirus infection, lower socioeconomic status, venereal diseases.

Pathology (major types)

Squamous cell carcinoma (90%), melanoma (5–6%), with adenocarcinoma, Paget's cell carcinoma, sarcoma, and verrucous carcinoma less than 1%.

Metastatic sites (major)

Pelvic and inguinal lymph nodes plus distant sites.

Associated malignancies

Cervical and vaginal cancer.

Therapy

Surgery, radiation, chemoradiation, and chemotherapy.

Recommendations to patient

Have venereal diseases treated promptly and have gynecological examinations at periodic intervals based on age and risk status. Any vulvar lesion that does not promptly respond to topical therapy should be considered for biopsy.

FOLLOW-UP OF THE PATIENT WITH VULVAR CANCER

	1st Year (Months)				2nd Year (Months)			3rd–5th Year (Months)		Thereafter (Months)
	3	6	9	12	4	8	12	6	12	12
History										
Complete				×			×		×	×
Bladder function	×	×	×		×	×		×		
Bone pain	×	×	×		×	×		×		
Bowel function	×	×	×		×	×		×		
Leg edema	×	×	×		×	×		×		
New vulvar lesion (mass, white area, ulcer)	×	×	×		×	×		×		
Physical										
Complete				×			×		×	×
Abdomen	×	×	×		×	×		×		
Breast	×	×	×		×	×		×		
Lymph nodes	×	×	×		×	×		×		
Pelvic exam	×	×	×		×	×		×		
Rectal	×	×	×		×	×		×		
Tests										
CBC		×		×			×		×	×
Chest x-ray				×			×			
Pap smear		×		×			×		×	×
Stool for blood				×			×		×	×
Urine				×			×		×	×

Comments: The patient must be an active partner in follow-up. She must be impressed with the need to return for examinations and to report promptly any new or persistent symptoms for the physician's evaluation. Nearly 80% of all recurrences may be expected within 3 years after definitive treatment, but some are seen at 5 years after therapy and later. Thus, lifelong follow-up on a regular progressed schedule is important.

8

BREAST CANCER

CONSULTANT: Monica Morrow, M.D.—Surgeon

The second most common malignancy in the United States and the second most common cause of cancer death in women (exceeded by lung cancer since 1986). Lifetime risk is 11% or 1 in 9.

INCIDENCE AND SURVIVAL

	Total	Male	Female
Incidence rate per 100,000/yr	59.5	0.9	108.4
Mortality rate per 100,000/yr	15.4	0.2	27.4
New cancer cases (ACS est 1994)	183,000	1,000	182,000
Cancer deaths (ACS est 1994)	46,300	300	46,000

5-year relative survival rates by stage

	Total	Under Age 50	Above Age 50
All stages	78.9%	77.0%	79.5%
Localized	93.1%	90.1%	94.3%
Regional	72.2%	69.4%	73.4%
Distant	18.2%	21.3%	17.5%
Unstaged	53.0%	59.5%	51.4%

Trends

Incidence is increasing slowly but mortality rates are constant, suggesting some improvement in survival associated with earlier diagnosis and better treatment.

Major risk factors

Older age, early menarche, late menopause, birth of first child after age 30, nulliparity, habitual alcohol consumption, radiation exposure (especially in childhood or adolescence). Family history in a first-degree relative (especially if premenopausal or bilateral). Cancer family syndromes (Li-Fraumeni syndrome, Cowden's disease, Muir syndrome). Atypical hyperplasia, lobular carcinoma in situ.

Pathology (major types)

Ductal (85% of cases), lobular, medullary, colloid, tubular, and papillary carcinomas.

Metastatic sites (major)

Regional lymph nodes (especially axillary, internal mammary, supraclavicular), lung, liver, bone, pleura, adrenals, and brain.

Associated malignancies

Colon, ovary, and endometrium.

Therapy

Surgery, radiation, hormones, and chemotherapy.

Recommendations to patient

Continue periodic screening for remaining breast tissue.

Recommendations to family

Obtain genetic counseling if first-degree relative with premenopausal cancer or multiple relatives are involved. Annual mammography beginning at age 40. If relatives had breast cancer before age 40, seek specific recommendations on age to begin mammography.

FOLLOW-UP OF THE PATIENT WITH BREAST CANCER

	First Year (Months)				2nd–5th Year (Months)		Thereafter (Months)
	3	6	9	12	6	12	12
History							
Complete				×		×	×
Lumps	×	×	×		×		
Cough, dyspnea	×	×	×		×		
Bone, chest pain	×	×	×		×		
Appetite, weight	×	×	×		×		
Breast self-exam	×	×	×		×		
Physical							
Complete				×		×	×
Mastectomy area	×	×	×		×		
Remaining breast	×	×	×		×		
Lymph nodes	×	×	×		×		
Abdomen, liver	×	×	×		×		
Chest	×	×	×		×		
Bones	×	×	×		×		
Tests							
Chest x-ray				×		×	×
CBC				×		×	×
Ca, LDH, Alk phos				×		×	×
Mammogram				×		×	×
Liver scan/CT or U/S	As indicated						
Bone scan	As indicated						

Comments: The scheme of follow-up should be individualized to reflect a patient's risk of recurrence. All women with one breast cancer are at increased risk for the development of a new contralateral primary tumor; this risk is approximately 1% per year. However, the risk of death from other primary tumors (ovary, endometrium, colon) is equal to or exceeds the risk of death from second primary breast cancer.[1] The role of routine laboratory and imaging studies to detect metastatic cancer when it is asymptomatic is controversial. A prospective, randomized trial[2] has demonstrated no survival benefit for routine testing compared to a careful history and physical exam with further studies directed by symptoms. The clinical role of tumor markers (CEA, CA 15-3) is unproven, and the use of these studies in follow-up will be elucidated by future research. Patients on tamoxifen should have periodic (at least yearly) gynecological examinations because of the increased incidence of endometrial carcinoma. Whether they need periodic ophthalmological examinations more often than the general age-matched population is unknown at this time. At present, the goal of salvage therapy is the relief of symptoms and the prolongation of survival. If advances in therapy result in more long-term survivors, the detection of clinically occult metastatic disease will be a worthwhile goal.

References

1. Rosen PP, Groshen S, Kinne DW, Norton L, Factors influencing prognosis in node negative breast carcinoma: Analysis of 767 T1N0M0/T2N0M0 patients with long term follow-up. J Clin Oncol 1993;11:2090.
2. Fossati R, Apolone G, Liberati A, et al., The effectiveness of follow-up diagnostic testing in patients with curable breast cancer: Results from a multi-center randomized trial. Proc Am Soc Clin Oncol 1994;13:77.

9 SKIN CANCERS

CUTANEOUS MELANOMA

CONSULTANTS: *Paul Calabresi, M.D.—Medical Oncologist*
Charles J.McDonald, M.D.—Dermatologist

Accounts for about 3% of all new cancer cases in the United States and is increasing along with increased sun exposure.

INCIDENCE AND SURVIVAL

	Total	Male	Female
Incidence rate per 100,000/yr	10.9	12.8	9.5
Mortality rate per 100,000/yr	2.2	3.0	1.5
New cancer cases (ACS est 1994)	32,000	17,000	15,000
Cancer deaths (ACS est 1994)	6900	4300	2600
5-year relative survival rates by stage			
All stages	84.1%	79.9%	88.6%
Localized	92.1%	89.7%	94.5%
Regional	54.6%	49.2%	62.3%
Distant	14.2%	10.7%	21.0%
Unstaged	61.2%	56.6%	66.6%

Trends

A 90% increase among whites from 1973 to 1990. The annual increase is 5% overall and 21% in young women. The highest increase of any cancer. The expected incidence by the year 2000 is 1 in 70–90 persons. Mortality is also increasing.

Major risk factors

Exposure to sun and other forms of ultraviolet radiation is a major cause. Family history, presence of dysplastic nevi, increased number of pigmented nevi.

Pathology (major types)

Superficial spreading melanoma, nodular melanoma, lentigo maligna melanoma, acral lentiginous melanoma, and unclassified type of melanoma.

Metastatic sites (major)

Local and regional sites in skin, regional lymph nodes, lung, liver, brain, bone, and intestines.

Associated malignancies

Basal and squamous cell carcinoma.

Therapy

Surgery, radiation, chemotherapy, and immunotherapy.

Recommendations to patient

Avoid excess exposure to sun and other sources of ultraviolet light. Use sunscreens, hats, protective clothing. Perform frequent skin examinations, self and professionally.

Recommendations to family

Avoid excess exposure to sun and other sources of ultraviolet light. Use sunscreens, hats, and protective clothing. Have skin checked periodically for suspicious lesions. Self-check every 3 months, professional every 6–12 months.

FOLLOW-UP OF THE PATIENT WITH CUTANEOUS MELANOMA

	1st Year (Months)				2nd–5th Year (Months)			Thereafter (Months)	
	3	6	9	12	4	8	12	6	12
History									
Complete				X		X	X		X
Skin	X	X	X		X	X		X	
Lumps	X	X	X		X	X		X	
GI symptoms	X	X	X		X	X		X	
CNS symptoms	X	X	X		X	X		X	
Pain	X	X	X		X	X		X	
Respiratory symptoms	X	X	X		X	X		X	
Physical									
Complete				X		X			X
Primary site	X	X	X		X	X		X	
Lymph nodes	X	X	X		X	X		X	
Chest	X	X	X		X	X		X	
Abdomen	X	X	X		X	X		X	
Liver	X	X	X		X	X		X	
Neurologic	X	X	X		X	X		X	
Skin	X	X	X		X	X		X	
Tests									
Chest x-ray				X		X			X
CBC	X	X	X	X	X	X	X	X	X
Liver function				X		X			X
Liver, bone, gallium scan	As indicated								
CT scan of brain	As indicated								

Comments: The natural history of melanoma is variable and depends to a significant degree on the clinical stage in which the tumor is detected. Therefore, any plan for follow-up of patients with melanoma should be individualized. The chart above should be considered a guide for follow-up of stage I disease, which does not involve local lymph nodes and is associated with substantial longevity. In such patients, tumor thickness and the presence or absence of a vertical growth phase is of fundamental importance. Eight-year survival of patients with stage I in the horizontal growth phase, irrespective of thickness, approximates 100%. Survival with stage II is at best 30–40% at 5 years and stage III approximates 6 months at best. Most recurrence is seen within 18 to 24 months. In general, local recurrence and regional lymph node involvement present earlier than in-transit metastasis, which itself presents earlier than distant metastasis. The most common sites of distant metastases are liver and lung; hence the need for chest x-rays and liver tests routinely. If a question of recurrence arises, a CT scan can be obtained to seek out the lesion. Accordingly, it is a good idea to obtain a baseline CT scan (if not already done) of the chest (lungs) and abdomen (liver) at the time of initial diagnosis for future comparison. Approximately 10% of patients with malignant melanoma have been found on follow-up examination and biopsy of dysplastic nevi to have a second primary melanoma; hence the need to examine the skin on the schedule basis above and to biopsy all suspicious lesions.

SKIN CANCER (NONMELANOMA)
CONSULTANT: Bijan Safai, M.D.—Dermatologist

The most common tumor site of all, so common that it is generally excluded from cancer statistics since it represents about 35% of all malignancies but has a very low mortality rate.

INCIDENCE AND SURVIVAL

	Total
Incidence rate per 100,000/yr	200
Mortality rate per 100,000/yr	0.6
5-year survival rate	
Basal cell carcinoma	99%
Squamous cell carcinoma	90%
New cancer cases (ACS est 1994)	700,000
Cancer deaths (ACS est 1994)	2300

Trends
Incidence increasing with increased leisure and inclination to spend much of it in activities in the sun, sometimes in the Sun Belt or in tanning salons.

Major risk factors
(1) Long-term sun exposure, (2) exposure to ionizing radiation, (3) arsenic, (4) presence of actinic keratoses, (5) xeroderma pigmentosum (recessive), (6) basal cell nevus syndrome (autosomal dominant), (7)human papillomavirus, (8) epidermodysplasia. Actinic keratosis by itself is a major precancerous condition and it may be caused by factors 1 and/or 2 and/or 3 listed here.

Pathology (major types)
Basal cell carcinoma (80%), squamous cell carcinoma (15–20%), and the remainder includes dermatofibrosarcoma protuberans and basal cell nevus syndrome.

Metastatic sites (major)
Regional lymph nodes, liver, and lung (mainly squamous cell, as basal cell carcinoma very rarely metastasizes).

Associated malignancies
Cutaneous melanoma, head and neck carcinoma.

Therapy
Curettage and electrodesiccation, surgery, radiation, chemotherapy, and cryosurgery.

Recommendations to patient
Avoid excessive sun exposure.

Recommendations to family
Obtain genetic counseling if hereditary types are diagnosed. Avoid excessive sun exposure.

FOLLOW-UP OF THE PATIENT WITH SKIN CANCER (NONMELANOMA)

	1st Year (Months)			2nd Year (Months)		Thereafter (Months)
	3	6	12	6	12	12
History						
Complete			×	×		×
Symptoms at lesion site	×	×		×		
Other lesions	×	×		×		
Physical						
Complete			×	×		×
Exam of lesion site	×	×		×		
Regional nodes	×	×		×		
Complete skin exam	×	×		×		
Tests						
Biopsy of new or recurrent lesion	As needed					

Comments: Basal cell carcinoma, also known as basal cell epithelioma, is a locally invasive destructive tumor that almost never metastasizes. The majority of these tumors are slow growing and may be present for several years before they become locally ulcerated and invasive and are recognized and correctly treated. A variety of therapies are available: surgical excision, electrodesiccation and curettage, or fractionated x-ray therapy. All are acceptable modes of therapy depending on the location and size of the lesion, age of the patient, and availability of therapies. Mohs' micrographic surgery is indicated for recurrent basal cell carcinoma and for primary tumors located in central facial areas such as alae nasi, and in periauricular areas. Consultation with a dermatologist versed in this cancer is recommended.

Squamous cell carcinomas arising from preceding actinic keratoses are locally invasive and rarely metastasize. Their malignant potential is considered less than that of squamous cell cancers arising on the lips, oral mucosa, or tongue. Squamous cell cancers arising in actinically damaged skin can be adequately treated by excision, fractionated x-ray, or Mohs' micrographic techniques depending on the size and location of the tumor, age of the patient, and availability of therapies. Lymph node biopsy is indicated only when regional palpable nodes are present.

KAPOSI'S SARCOMA (KS)—CLASSICAL AND AIDS RELATED

CONSULTANTS: Alvin E. Friedman-Kien, M.D.—Dermatologist
Abraham Chachoua, M.D.—Medical Oncologist

Classical Kaposi's sarcoma (CKS) represents a rare, indolent tumor usually appearing on the skin of the lower extremities in a bilateral symmetrical distribution. The disease occurs predominantly in elderly men of Eastern European or Mediterranean origin, with the male:female ratio about 15:1. It is not usually associated with immune suppression and tends to remain localized to the skin on the lower extremities, occasionally with local invasion of subcutaneous tissue and bone. Involvement of internal organs does not usually occur. Patients with CKS usually remain relatively asymptomatic and may require no therapy for several years. As the tumors gradually increase in size and new lesions develop over several years, lymphatic involvement may cause considerable lymphedema of the lower extremities.

In Central Africa where KS has long been recognized to be a common endemic disease in the absence of HIV infection, predominantly seen in males, it accounts for 10% of all neoplastic diseases reported in that region. It may be seen both as an indolent and as a "classical" type and as a more aggressive form of KS with cutaneous and lymph node involvement, in which local invasion of the subcutaneous tissue and bone is frequently observed.

Follow-up of patients with CKS depends on the symptomatic nature of their disease. In most cases the skin lesions remain asymptomatic for long periods. As the skin lesions tend to slowly enlarge, they become nodular and ulcerated, and often become secondarily infected. They may become painful, especially when associated with chronic lymphedema of the involved extremities. Such patients should be examined approximately every 2–4 months for reevaluation depending on the extent of clinical symptoms. As the disease becomes symptomatic, patients should be seen more frequently depending on the type of treatment chosen by the physician.

Tests should include CBC, blood chemistries, and parameters of immune functions, especially the peripheral blood (CD4) T-lymphocyte count and an HIV antibody on initial examination because even the aged are HIV infection susceptible.

Treatment of individual CKS lesions ranges from local cryotherapy, radiation therapy, and surgical excision to intralesional injections of chemotherapeutic agents such as vinblastine, which have proven to be effective in providing palliation of the smaller skin KS lesions. The systemic administration of single and/or combinations of chemotherapeutic agents such as bleomycin, vincristine, and adriamycin has been found to be palliative for varying lengths of time. Systemic treatment with liposome-encapsulated doxorubicin is under evaluation for CKS, especially in those patients whose tumors have become resistant to the traditional chemotherapeutic agents.

FOLLOW-UP OF THE PATIENT WITH AIDS-ASSOCIATED KAPOSI'S SARCOMA

In contrast to CKS, patients with AIDS-KS are generally much more ill with a clinical picture dominated by the underlying, profound immune suppression characteristic of HIV disease as manifested by the various opportunistic infections to which these patients are prone. The KS tumor lesions in these individuals are much more aggressive and widely disseminated than with CKS. The patients tend to develop multiple remarkably symmetrical, patch, plaque, and nodular lesions of the skin and oral mucosa often with involvement of the lymph nodes, gastrointestinal tract, lungs, and other visceral organs. Evaluation should include a full history and physical examination with particular attention to the oral cavity, lymph nodes, and lungs, periodic chest x-ray, CBC, chemistries, and (CD4) T-lymphocyte determinations. Progression of AIDS-KS usually occurs as the CD4 count drops below 100. CT scans of the chest may be helpful if pulmonary involvement is suspected.

The recommended follow-up for patients with asymptomatic AIDS-KS includes monthly visits with particular attention to the size of individual lesions or an increase in the number of new lesions or the development of troublesome symptoms such as edema of an involved extremity, the head, and neck due to lymphatic obstruction as well as secondary bacterial infection with erosion of the larger, nodular skin lesions.

The treatment of AIDS-KS depends on the extent and severity of clinical disease as well as the location of the lesions, which are often cosmetically disturbing. Local cryotherapy with liquid nitrogen, intralesional injections with diluted chemotherapeutic agents like vinblastine, and radiation therapy can be very effective for treating individual skin lesions. As the disease becomes more widely disseminated, repeated administration of systemic chemotherapy with interferon alpha, or single and combination antineoplastic agents including vincristine, bleomycin, and doxorubicin (Adriamycin), have been shown to be beneficial. In addition, liposome-encapsulated anthracyclines (doxorubicin or daunorubicin) have been found to be useful in patients with AIDS-KS in whom the disease has ceased to respond to standard chemotherapy.

Follow-up laboratory examinations should include a monthly CBC and blood chemistries to detect anemia or other abnormalities that may be suggestive of visceral involvement. The absolute CD4 count should be performed in the HIV-positive individual every 3–4 months. Patients receiving chemotherapy are usually seen more frequently. Such patients are usually examined every 1–3 weeks, depending on the chemotherapeutic regimen used. It should be emphasized that AIDS-KS is usually fatal as a consequence of pulmonary involvement.

10

OSTEOSARCOMA
CONSULTANT: Henry J. Mankin, M.D.—Surgeon

A malignant spindle cell tumor that produces osteoid and is the most common primary malignant adult bone tumor (with the exception of multiple myeloma, which is usually grouped with the hematopoietic malignancies).

INCIDENCE AND SURVIVAL

	Total	Male	Female
Incidence rate per 100,000/yr	0.2		
Mortality rate per 100,000/yr	0.2		
New bone cancer cases (est 1994)	2000	1100	900
New osteosarcoma cases (est 1994)	1000	550	450
Bone cancer deaths (est 1994)	1075	600	475
2-year survival rates by stage			
Localized	40–90%		
Distant	30–60%		

Trends
Incidence stable. Mortality decreased since survival improved.

Major risk factors
Familial retinoblastoma (rare), other oncogenic abnormalities (eg, p53), ionizing radiation, Paget's disease, rapid bone growth (as in adolescence and in areas of trauma).

Pathology (major types)
Classic osteogenic sarcoma (with malignant spindle cells, stroma, and osteoid formation), fibroblastic, parosteal, chondroblastic, periosteal, and telangiectatic osteogenic sarcoma. Malignant fibrous histiocytoma and fibrosarcoma of bone are similar and may be identical malignancies.

Metastatic sites (major)
Lung and bone.

Associated malignancies
Retinoblastoma (rarely).

Therapy
Surgery (including limb salvage), adjuvant chemotherapy, and less commonly, radiation.

Recommendations to patient
Report cough or pulmonary symptoms or local pain to physician promptly.

Recommendations to family
Obtain genetic counseling if familial or retinoblastoma associated.

FOLLOW-UP OF THE PATIENT WITH OSTEOSARCOMA

	1st Year (Months)						2nd Year (Months)				3rd and 4th Year (Months)				Thereafter (Months)
	2	4	6	8	10	12	3	6	9	12	4	6	8	12	12
History															
Complete						×				×				×	×
Pain	×	×	×	×	×		×	×	×		×		×		
Mass	×	×	×	×	×		×	×	×		×		×		
Appetite, weight	×	×	×	×	×		×	×	×		×		×		
Respiratory	×	×	×	×	×		×	×	×		×		×		
CNS	×	×	×	×	×		×	×	×		×		×		
Distal neurovascular	×	×	×	×	×		×	×	×		×		×		
Physical															
Complete						×				×				×	×
Primary site	×	×	×	×	×		×	×	×		×		×		
Lymph nodes	×	×	×	×	×		×	×	×		×		×		
Chest	×	×	×	×	×		×	×	×		×		×		
Distal neurovascular	×	×	×	×	×		×	×	×		×		×		
Abdomen	×	×	×	×	×		×	×	×		×		×		
Tests															
Chest x-ray	×	×	×	×	×	×	×	×	×	×	×		×	×	×
CT of chest		×		×		×		×		×		×		×	×
Bone scan		×		×		×				×				×	×
X-ray of primary site	×	×	×	×	×	×	×	×	×	×	×		×	×	×
CBC	×	×	×	×	×	×	×	×	×	×	×			×	×
Liver function	×	×	×	×	×	×	×	×	×	×	×			×	×
Serum creatinine	×	×	×	×	×	×	×	×	×	×	×			×	×
Additional tests	As indicated														

Comments: Patients should be followed closely with serial imaging studies looking for local recurrence or distant metastases. As a general rule, they should be seen every 2 months for the first year with chest x-rays and a CT of the chest and bone scan at 4 and 8 months. The time interval for visits is 3 months in the second year, 4 months in the third and fourth years, and 6 months to 1 year thereafter. Chest x-rays and x-rays of the primary site should be obtained at each visit (especially for patients who have had limb-sparing surgery) and a chest CT every 6 months until the fourth year, then yearly. A bone scan should be obtained yearly. Liver and kidney function tests are important during chemotherapy and for 2 years afterward. The serum alkaline phosphatase is sometimes elevated with local recurrence or metastases.

EWING'S SARCOMA

CONSULTANTS: Gerald Rosen, M.D.—Medical and Pediatric Oncologist

Gary E. Friedlaender, M.D.—Orthopedic Oncologic Surgeon

Ewing's sarcoma is a rare tumor of bone that affects both the long bones and the flat bones (pelvis, scapula, and spine) of patients predominantly under age 30. Lesions in the pelvis or spine can present as low back pain and are sometimes mistaken for "disc" disease. Persistent pain in a patient under age 30 should lead to either a bone scan, a CT scan of the pelvic area or spine, or a simple x-ray of an involved long bone. When a suspicious lesion is identified, it should be confirmed by biopsy. Ewing's sarcoma is a highly malignant tumor the treatment of which is greatly benefited by the use of chemotherapy. Radiation therapy (RT) is used to control the primary tumor; however, it is imperative that surgical resection of the lesional area be done following preoperative RT and chemotherapy since there is a high incidence (>25%) of late local recurrences in the primary site following high-dose RT alone without surgical resection of the primary lesion. Some institutions do not use radiation therapy if a primary curative resection is feasible. This avoids the risk of radiation-induced sarcoma.

INCIDENCE AND SURVIVAL

	Total
Incidence rate per 100,000/yr	0.17
5-year survival rates by stage	
All stages	50%
Localized	50–70%
Distant	20–45%

Trends

Incidence decrease may be apparent due to classification changes by pathologists. Mortality decreased since survival improved.

Pathology (major types)

Uniform sheets of small round blue cells with indistinct cytoplasmic borders and small round nuclei. Seen primarily in diaphysis of long bones and in flat bones (pelvis, scapula, ribs, and vertebral bodies). Recent evidence suggests that the tumor is derived from neural tissue and not endothelial cells. Its chromosomal translocation is indistinguishable from peripheral neuroepithelioma (primitive neuroectodermal tumor [PNET]).

Metastatic sites (major)

Lung, bone, bone marrow, and CNS.

Therapy

Chemotherapy, radiation therapy, and limb salvage surgery.

Recommendations to patient

Report pain, cough, or pulmonary symptoms to physician promptly.

FOLLOW-UP OF THE PATIENT WITH EWING'S SARCOMA

	1st Year (Months)				2nd Year (Months)				3rd–7th Year (Months)		Thereafter (Months)
	3	6	9	12	4	6	8	12	6	12	12
History											
Complete				×				×		×	×
Pain	×	×	×		×		×		×		
Mass	×	×	×		×		×		×		
Appetite, weight	×	×	×		×		×		×		
Respiratory	×	×	×		×		×		×		
CNS	×	×	×		×		×		×		
Physical											
Complete				×				×		×	×
Primary site	×	×	×		×		×		×		
Regional lymph nodes	×	×	×		×		×		×		
Chest	×	×	×		×		×		×		
Abdomen	×	×	×		×		×		×		
Tests											
CT scan of chest	×	×	×	×	×		×	×	×	×	×
X-ray of primary site	×	×	×	×	×		×	×	×	×	×
Bone scan	×	×	×	×		×		×	×	×	×
CT/MRI of primary site		×		×		×		×	×	×	×
CBC		×		×	×			×	×	×	×
Liver function	As indicated										
Additional specific	As indicated										

Comments: Follow-up studies in patients who have completed multimodality treatment, including chemotherapy, preoperative radiation therapy, and surgical resection of the tumor (which is usually followed by more chemotherapy), should include a CT scan of the lungs done every 3 months for the first year after completion of chemotherapy, every 4 months for the second year, and then every 6 months for the next 5 years. In addition, imaging studies of the primary tumor area should be done if it has not been completely surgically resected. The most useful imaging studies in local follow-up of Ewing's sarcoma are CT/MRI scans, which can detect bony as well as soft-tissue abnormalities. Different institutions and radiologists select one or the other depending on what is their primary imaging concern diagnostically. Chest x-rays are infrequently used now since the CT scan provides so much more definitive information about the status of the lungs. Bone scan should be done every 3 months for the first year off chemotherapy and then every 6 months for the next 3–4 years. The most frequent symptom of a recurrence is pain in a bone, which should be followed up with appropriate imaging studies. Pulmonary recurrences are usually not symptomatic but the above schedule of chest CT scans should be sufficient to detect recurrent disease. The two most important variables for a good prognosis include complete surgical resection of the primary lesional area and chemotherapy with high doses of active agents like ifosfamide (with mesna) and doxorubicin.

ADULT SOFT TISSUE SARCOMA

CONSULTANT: Steven A. Rosenberg, M.D.—Surgeon

Accounts for 0.7% of new cases of cancer and 0.6% of cancer deaths in the United States. With improved combined modality therapy, survival is improving and limb-sparing procedures are now feasible and successful.

INCIDENCE AND SURVIVAL

	Total	Male	Female
Incidence rate per 100,000/yr	2.1	2.5	1.7
Mortality rate per 100,000/yr	1.1	1.2	1.2
5-year survival rate	61.5%	59.3%	64.2%
New cancer cases (ACS est 1994)	6000	3300	2700
Cancer deaths (ACS est 1994)	3300	1600	1700
5-year survival rates by stage			
Stage I	>90%		
Stage II	70%		
Stage III	20–50%		
Stage IV	<20%		

Major risk factors

Von Recklinghausen's neurofibromatosis.

Pathology (major types)

Malignant fibrous histiocytoma, fibrosarcoma, mesenchymoma, liposarcoma, rhabdomyosarcoma, synovial cell sarcoma, epithelial sarcoma, angiosarcoma, lymphangiosarcoma, hemangiopericytoma, malignant schwannoma, neuroepithelioma, alveolar soft-part sarcoma.

Metastatic sites (major)

Lung.

Therapy

Surgery, radiation, and chemotherapy.

Recommendations to patient

Have new lumps that increase in size or persist more than 3 weeks checked by a physician.

FOLLOW-UP OF THE PATIENT WITH BONE AND SOFT TISSUE SARCOMAS

	1st–5th Year (Months)		Thereafter (Months)
	6	12	12
History			
Complete	×	×	×
Pain			
Mass			
Appetite, weight			
Respiratory			
CNS			
Distal neurovascular			
Physical			
Complete	×	×	×
Primary site			
Regional lymph nodes			
Chest			
Distal neurovascular			
Abdomen			
Tests			
Chest x-ray	×	×	×
CT of chest		×	
CT/MRI of primary site		×	
CBC		×	
Liver function		×	
Other tests	As indicated		

Comments: Primary soft tissue tumors, while rare, affect the extremities and trunk in individuals of all ages. Because of their infrequent nature, these neoplasms are often misdiagnosed, confused with other benign diseases, or overlooked. Limb-sparing tumor resections are often feasible, following accurate diagnostic biopsy (needle or open) and staging. Like primary bone and cartilage tumors, these lesions often benefit from combined surgical, chemotherapeutic, and irradiation approaches. Also, like skeletal tumors, these malignancies tend to metastasize to the lung. Unlike primary osseous tumors, plain x-rays are often unrewarding, but the use of CT or MRI scans, angiography, and other selected diagnostic imaging approaches offer excellent resolution of local disease. Close follow-up is important, since aggressive surgical treatment of lung metastases has been associated with substantial long-term survival.

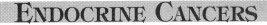

ENDOCRINE CANCERS

THYROID CANCER

CONSULTANT: William M. McConahey, M.D.—Endocrinologist

This malignancy accounts for 1% of all cancers diagnosed and is usually more common in females. Of the five types of thyroid carcinoma described, papillary cancer comprises approximately 75% of the cases, follicular 9%, Hürthle-cell variant of follicular 2%, medullary (both sporadic and familial) 6%, and anaplastic 8%. The risk of developing papillary or follicular thyroid carcinoma is increased in those persons who have had radiation therapy to the tonsils and adenoids (a procedure once considered to be useful and safe but no longer employed). A similar correlation is present with patients irradiated to the mediastinum during infancy to prevent the so-called status thymolymphaticus that was thought at one time to be the cause of sudden crib deaths in infants.

INCIDENCE AND SURVIVAL

Overall statistics including all groups	Total	Male	Female
Incidence rate per 100,000/yr	4.5	2.5	6.4
Mortality rate per 100,000/yr	0.3	0.3	0.4
New cancer cases (ACS est 1994)	13,000	3,400	9,600
Cancer deaths (ACS est 1994)	1,025	400	625

Mean age at diagnoses: papillary, 44 years; follicular, 53 years; medullary, 51 years; anaplastic, 65 years. Of papillary thyroid carcinoma, 15–20% are diagnosed before age 30.

Sex variation: In all types of thyroid carcinoma, except the anaplastic, the disease is approximately twice as common in females as in males. Anaplastic carcinoma occurs about twice as often in males as in females.

5-year survival rates for the histologic types of thyroid carcinoma

Type of Malignancy	All stages	Localized	Regional	Distant
Papillary	97%	99%	95%	45%
Follicular	90%	98%	73%	40%
Medullary	79%	96%	70%	25%
Anaplastic	3.5%	0%	0%	0%

Major risk factors

Ionizing radiation, discrete nodules in thyroid or neck, goiters, possibly iodine deficiency or prolonged TSH stimulation of high degree, and familial history of multiple endocrine neoplasia (cases of medullary carcinoma).

Metastatic sites (major)

Lung, bone, mediastinum, regional lymph nodes, and liver.

Therapy

Surgery for all but completely inoperable cases; postoperative radioiodine therapy for selected papillary or follicular carcinomas (those having significant functioning residual thyroid tissue or metastases remaining after surgery); external radiation for bone, lung, or mediastinal metastases that do not pick up enough radioiodine for effective therapy; and suppression of TSH by the administration of levothyroxine. Chemotherapy is rarely helpful.

Recommendations to patient

Report to physician promptly if new nodules are felt in the neck, and have follow-up with endocrinologist in addition to oncologist.

Recommendations to family

Obtain physician examination if a relative develops medullary thyroid cancer or multiple endocrine neoplasia syndrome.

FOLLOW-UP OF THE PATIENT WITH THYROID CANCER

	1st Year (Months)			2nd–5th Year (Months)		Thereafter (Months)
	1	6	12	6	12	12
History						
Complete			X		X	X
Cough, hoarseness	X	X		X		
Lumps	X	X		X		
Muscle spasm	X	X		X		
Bone pain	X	X		X		
Thyroid symptoms	X	X		X		
Physical						
Complete			X		X	X
Operative site	X	X		X		
Neck	X	X		X		
Chest	X	X		X		
Abdomen	X	X		X		
Tests						
Chest x-ray	X	X	X		X	X
CBC	X	X	X		X	X
Thyroid scan	X		X			
Thyroglobulin	X	X	X		X	X
Bone scan	If indicated by pain					
Special endocrine	For medullary carcinoma					

Comments: The best test for the diagnosis of carcinoma in a thyroid nodule is the fine-needle aspiration biopsy of the nodule. A valuable laboratory test for the diagnosis of medullary carcinoma is basal and stimulated concentration of calcitonin.

Prognosis in thyroid carcinoma is closely related to histologic type. The longest survivals are associated with well-differentiated papillary carcinoma, but it can recur and it can kill. Follicular carcinoma and medullary carcinoma are not as indolent but have a reasonably good prognosis. Poorly differentiated or anaplastic thyroid carcinomas have a very poor prognosis with a rapid growth, dissemination, and early death in almost all cases. Total-body 131-iodine scans are helpful in follow-up of patients with papillary or follicular tumors, especially if a total thyroidectomy has been performed. Replacement levothyroxine should be discontinued before 131-iodine scan. An endocrinologist should participate in the management and follow-up. The technetium bone scan is also useful if the patient has bone pain or there is any other reason to suspect bone metastases.

Thyroglobulin levels, when elevated, are diagnostic of local or metastatic spread. Thyroglobulin is more likely to be elevated in a hypothyroid patient, but it may be increased in euthyroid patients. For localized metastatic disease, CT scan or MRI scan is often very useful.

ISLET CELL NEOPLASIA

CONSULTANT: Irvin M. Modlin, M.D.,Ph.D.—Endocrine Surgeon/Physiologist

A tumor of the islet cells of the pancreas. Found in 1–1.5% of autopsy series. Clinical symptomatology often mundane; therefore, clinical diagnosis sometimes difficult. Recognition of the characteristic syndrome facilitates diagnosis, particularly if appropriate plasma peptides and amines are measured. The tumors may be functional due to oversecretion of a specific hormone. Between 70% and 80% of such lesions are benign. Some may, however, be multicentric within the pancreas. Nonfunctional lesions can be relatively benign, but often represent a far more malignant pattern than their functional counterparts.

INCIDENCE AND SURVIVAL

	Total
Incidence rate per 100,000/yr	0.1–0.4
5-year relative survival rate	
For Gastrinoma	65%
For Insulinoma	60%
New cancer cases (est 1994)	200–1000

BIOCHEMICAL PATHOLOGY

Islet cell	Secretion	Tumor—Syndrome
Alpha	Glucagon	Glucagonoma—diabetes, dermatitis
Beta	Insulin	Insulinoma—hypoglycemia
Delta	Somatostatin	Somatostatinoma—diabetes, mild
D	Gastrin	Gastrinoma—peptic ulcer disease
A–D	Vasoactive intestinal peptide (VIP)	WDHA—watery diarrhea, hypokalemic acidosis (VIPoma)
	5-HT	Carcinoid
	ACTH	Cushing's disease
	MSH	Hyperpigmentation
Interacinar cells		
F	Pancreatic polypeptide	Multiple hormonal syndromes
EC	5-HT (serotonin)	Carcinoid

Major risk factors

Familial cancer syndrome (MEN-I [multiple endocrine neoplasia, type I]).

Metastatic sites (major)

Peritoneum, regional lymph nodes, liver, and bone.

Associated malignancies

Parathyroid, thyroid, adrenal, and pancreas.

Therapy

Surgery, chemotherapy, hormonal therapy, and immunotherapy.

Recommendations to patient

Request physician to give symptom therapy as needed.

Recommendations to family

Obtain genetic counseling if hereditary influence such as MEN is involved.

FOLLOW-UP OF THE PATIENT WITH ISLET CELL NEOPLASIA

	1st Year (Months)				2nd–5th Year (Months)				Thereafter (Months)	
	3	6	9	12	3	6	9	12	6	12
History										
Complete				×				×		×
Dyspepsia	×	×	×		×	×	×			
Diarrhea	×	×	×		×	×	×			
Sweating	×	×	×		×	×	×			
Fainting	×	×	×		×	×	×			
Skin rash	×	×	×		×	×	×			
Flushing	×	×	×		×	×	×			
Wheezing	×	×	×		×	×	×			
Weight loss	×	×	×		×	×	×			
Physical										
Complete				×				×		×
Lymph nodes	×	×	×		×					
Chest	×	×	×		×					
Abdominal masses	×	×	×		×					
Liver	×	×	×		×					
Rectal	×	×	×		×					
Tests										
Plasma peptides/amines	×	×	×	×		×		×	×	×
Urine 5-HIAA		×		×		×		×	×	×
Chest x-ray		×		×	×			×		
CT scan of abdomen or MRI (STIR)*				×				×		
Octreoscan				×				×		
Panendoscopy				×				×		

*STIR MRI = spin tau inversion recovery magnetic resonance imaging.

Comments: Islet cell tumors of the pancreas are rare and are often diagnosed late because their mundane symptoms may not suggest a neoplastic process. Recurrence of the tumor is usually at a local site in the retroperitoneum, in lymph nodes, and the liver. Clinical diagnosis is best made by the recrudescence of the symptomatology with which the patient originally presented. Prior to such manifestations, measurement of the relevant peptide or amine in the plasma is an earlier indication of tumor regrowth. Topographical localization is best obtained using either a radioisotope study (octreoscan) or else MRI or CT scan. Conventional x-ray techniques or ultrasound are relatively insensitive in detecting the recurrence of such lesions. Topographic localization of tumor recurrence may be difficult due to previous surgery interfering with image reconstruction and interpretation. Although cure of metastases is seldom possible, substantial relief of symptoms from excessive hormonal polypeptides is usually possible by use of blocking agents.

ADRENOCORTICAL CARCINOMA
CONSULTANT: Philip K. Bondy, M.D.—Endocrinologist

A malignant neoplasm of adrenal cortical cells with partial or complete histological and functional differentiation. Comprises only 0.05–0.2% of all cancers. Ten percent are associated with masculinization and 12% with feminization. Many functioning tumors cause hypokalemic alkalosis. The endocrine pattern can change during the course of the tumor.

INCIDENCE AND SURVIVAL

	Total
Incidence rate per 100,000/yr	0.2
5-year survival rate	20%
5-year survival rates by stage	
Stage I	80%
Stage II	50%
Stage III	20–30%
Stage IV	1–5%

Major risk factors

In cushingoid patients, impaired immune response, diabetes, hypokalemic alkalosis, and increased risk of osteoporosis.

Pathology (major types)

Malignant adenocarcinoma with cells with big nuclei, hyperchromatism, increased numbers of mitoses, and enlarged nucleoli. Some cancers (especially in children) may appear to be benign.

Metastatic sites (major)

Regional lymph nodes and adjacent organs such as liver, kidney, diaphragm, and pancreas. Lung, bone, and mesentery are also often involved.

Associated malignancies

Breast and lung carcinomas, soft tissue sarcomas.

Therapy

Surgery is preferred. Radiation is seldom useful. Hormonal treatment may be needed to support failing secretion (especially of corticosteroids) caused by treatment. Chemotherapy directed at suppressing steroid secretion may relieve cushingoid symptoms. Response to chemotherapy for tumor suppression is usually temporary and limited.

Recommendations to patient

Report infections without delay because of suppressed immune function. Instruct patients receiving mitotane, aminoglutethimide, metyrapone, ketoconazole, or combinations to report symptoms of adrenal failure.

Recommendations to family

Obtain genetic counseling if there is evidence of hereditary patterns.

FOLLOW-UP OF THE PATIENT WITH ADRENOCORTICAL CARCINOMA

	1st Year (Months)				2nd–5th Year (Months)		Thereafter (Months)
	1	4	8	12	6	12	12
History							
Complete				×		×	×
Abdominal pain or fullness	×	×	×		×		
Abdominal masses	×	×	×		×		
Virilization in female	×	×	×		×		
Feminization in male	×	×	×		×		
Symptoms of alkalosis (eg, tetany)	×	×	×		×		
Unexplained weight loss	×	×	×		×		
Unexplained fever	×	×	×		×		
Physical							
Complete				×		×	×
Operative site	×	×	×		×		
Chest	×	×	×		×		
Abdomen	×	×	×		×		
Cushingoid features	×	×	×		×		
Hirsutism (female or child)	×	×	×		×		
Gynecomastia (male or child)	×	×	×		×		
Tetany	×	×	×		×		
Tests							
Chest x-ray	×	×	×	×		×	×
CBC	×	×	×	×		×	×
CT or MRI of abdomen		×	×	×		×	
Blood chemistries, ie, glucose electrolytes	×	×	×	×	×	×	×
Urinary steroids (DHEA if masculinized; 17-hydroxysteroids or tetrahydrocortisone if cushingoid)		×	×	×		×	×
Plasma cortisol, DHEA, estrogens according to symptoms	×	×	×	×	×	×	

Comments: Only about half of patients with adrenocortical carcinoma have endocrine symptoms, which may vary as the disease progresses. Adrenocortical cancers of infants and children often appear benign histologically but are extremely difficult to cure surgically. Most functioning tumors secrete excessive amounts of deoxycorticosterone and therefore cause hypokalemic alkalosis. Nonfunctioning tumors present with abdominal pain, a sensation of fullness, or an abdominal mass. Some are found incidentally during x-ray examination. Surgery is the only hope for cure. Agents suppressing corticosteroid secretion (mitotane, aminoglutethimide, metyrapone, ketoconazole) may provide relief from cushingoid symptoms and, indeed, may cause life-endangering adrenocortical insufficiency unless corticosteroid treatment is given. Chemotherapy with mitotane sometimes causes complete remission; cisplatin, etoposide, doxorubicin, and melphalan may produce partial remission, but chemotherapy seldom prolongs life.

Metastases from tumors of the lung and breast frequently occur in the adrenal, usually bilaterally, but must be distinguished from primary tumor if unilateral.

PHEOCHROMOCYTOMA (PCC)
CONSULTANT: Philip K. Bondy, M.D.—Endocrinologist

A rare tumor of chromaffin cells arising from the adrenal medulla in 90% of cases, and from extra-adrenal chromaffin tissue in the remainder. Ten percent are bilateral, primarily in familial cases associated with the multiple endocrine neoplasia (MEN) syndrome, types II A, II B, and III. Incidence of malignancy ranges from 5% to 46%. Extra-adrenal tumors are more likely to be malignant. Although only 0.1–0.5% of hypertensive patients have PCC, early recognition is important since >90% of PCC patients are cured with treatment. The hypertension may be sustained or paroxysmal, is often severe, sometimes with encephalopathy, retinopathy, and proteinuria. Untreated patients run a high risk of sudden death.

INCIDENCE AND SURVIVAL

	Total
New tumor cases (est 1994)	800
5-year relative survival rates by stage	
Localized, benign	>95%
Regional	No hard data (probably ±75%)
Distant	40% (32–60%)

Major risk factors

Malignant hypertension or congestive heart failure is the usual cause of death. Association with medullary thyroid cancer in MEN type II A and II B carries additional risk from associated tumors. Also occurs in 25% of patients with Lindau–von Hippel disease, 1% of patients with neurofibromatosis and von Recklinghausen's disease.

Pathology (major types)

Arises from chromaffin cells in sympathetic neural ganglia and the adrenal medulla. The tumors produce catecholamines which cause hypertension and its complications. Mixed tumors can produce ACTH and corticosteroids, causing Cushing's syndrome. They can also make peptide hormones, eg, oxytocin, vasopressin, somatostatin, and calcitonin, but these are seldom clinically significant.

Metastatic sites (major)

Regional infiltration; lymph nodes, bones, liver, and lungs.

Associated syndromes

Cerebellar hemangioblastoma, Sturge-Weber syndrome, and tuberous sclerosis.

Therapy

Surgery is the only curative procedure. Radiation and chemotherapy are ineffective. Control of symptoms of hypertension is essential preoperatively and symptomatically helpful during recurrences of metastatic cancer.

Recommendations to patient

Cooperate in control of hypertension. Report masses, pain, etc, for possible local treatment.

Recommendations to family

Seek genetic counseling in families with MEN or other familial history.

FOLLOW-UP OF THE PATIENT WITH PHEOCHROMOCYTOMA

	1st Year (Months)		Thereafter (Months)
	6	12	12
History			
Complete		X	X
Anxiety attacks	X		
Paroxysmal headaches	X		
Palpitations	X		
Diaphoresis	X		
Weight	X		
Physical			
Complete		X	X
Blood pressure	X		
Orthostatic hypotension	X		
Abdominal mass	X		
Tests			
Urine catecholamines	X	X	X
Catechol, metabolites		X	X
Chest x-ray		X	X
Abdominal CT or MRI		X	As indicated

Comments: The objective of initial treatment for pheochromocytoma, whether benign or malignant, is to correct hypertension. Patients therefore need the usual surgical follow-up and close observation of blood pressure and renal function. Because it is impossible to make a secure distinction between benign and malignant pheochromocytomas by histology, further follow-up is required, as indicated in the chart. Recurrences in the 10% of malignant tumors usually are within 5 to 6 years, but may appear after 20 years. Monitoring the blood pressure is therefore essential for the remainder of the patient's life. Catecholamine determinations are indicated after the first 2 years only if the blood pressure begins to rise again. If there is evidence of recurrence, CT scan or MRI are the best methods of determining location and extent of the tumor. Scintigraphy with 131-I-meta-iodobenzylguanidine (131-I-MIBG) may help. Surgical excision of the primary tumor is the only successful approach. Excision of isolated large metastases may give symptomatic relief. Radiation and chemotherapy are of limited value. Therapeutic doses of 131-I-MIBG are sometimes said to help. Since the tumor grows very slowly, the most important symptomatic benefit occurs with control of hypertension with phenoxybenzamine, propranolol, and alpha-methyl-p-tyrosine (metyrosine) to block synthesis of catecholamines. Corticosteroid support will be necessary after bilateral adrenalectomy. Symptomatic support may permit patients with metastases to survive many years.

12

CARCINOMA OF UNKNOWN PRIMARY (CUP)

CONSULTANT: John E. Ultmann, M.D.—Medical Oncologist

Accounts for about 5–10% of all cancer patients. These patients have biopsy proven cancer presenting as metastases, and after reasonable evaluation with history, physical examination, standard laboratory tests, and chest x-ray, no primary site is identified. An identification of the primary is sometimes possible with more extensive diagnostic imaging, usually CT scan of the abdomen, pelvis, and/or chest. Sometimes identification results from special histologic processing, eg, immunoperoxidases, estrogen or progesterone receptors, electron micrography, or tumor markers, eg, prostate specific antigen (PSA), alpha-fetoprotein (AFP), or beta–human chorionic gonadotropin (beta-HCG). About 15–25% remain undiagnosed as to primary source even at autopsy.

INCIDENCE AND SURVIVAL

	Total
Incidence rate per 100,000/yr	24.5
Mortality rate per 100,000/yr	close to incidence
5-year relative survival rate	<10%
New cancer cases (est 1994)	45,000–70,000
Cancer deaths (est 1994)	no data available

Survival duration

No reliable mortality or survival statistics are available at the present time. This is a heterogeneous group of patients that had been assumed to be aged, undiagnosable, and unresponsive to therapy. More recently, the diagnosis has also included a younger cohort of patients, mostly males with CUP in the mediastinum and retroperitoneum with negative AFP and beta-HCG, who have responded to therapy with cisplatin-based chemotherapy regimens; it is estimated that 10–15% of all CUP falls into this group, accounting for 5000 patients annually. In addition, when certain specific primaries are finally identified, eg, lymphoma, breast, prostate, germ cell carcinomas, and Ewing's sarcoma, appropriate therapy often results in improved survival and occasional cures.

Pathology (major types)

Poorly differentiated neoplasms, some with characteristics of adenocarcinoma, squamous cell carcinoma, or just poorly differentiated cancer; even when the primary is ultimately identified the tumor is more anaplastic than the usual type.

Metastatic sites (major)

Retroperitoneum, mediastinum, other lymph node areas, liver, lung, bone, brain, meninges, and skin.

Therapy

Surgery, chemotherapy, and radiation.

FOLLOW-UP OF THE PATIENT WITH CARCINOMA OF UNKNOWN PRIMARY (CUP)

CUP is a heterogeneous group of cancers. Appropriate limited work-up may have led to a definitive or strongly presumptive diagnosis and consequent "appropriate" therapy.

When and if a definitive diagnosis is made, more precise therapy can be given, as described in standard texts (see Bibliography). Then the follow-up can also be more precise, and with the diagnosis, one should seek the relevant section for follow-up recommendations, which are likely to be for head and neck, lung, pancreas, atypical germ cell tumors, testicular cancer, etc. Occult primary metastatic (squamous cell) neck cancers are discussed separately on page 24.

For patients in whom no diagnosis can be established but who have the highest statistical chance to have a primary in the lung (above-diaphragm presentation of adenocarcinoma or squamous cell carcinoma), consult the section on non–small-cell lung cancer; or in the pancreas (below-diaphragm presentation of adenocarcinoma), consult the pancreatic cancer section.

Follow-up must address:
1. Occurrence of pain and its diagnosis and treatment
2. Complications of tumor mass(es) or metastasis or of eventual growth of the primary tumor
3. Recognition of paraneoplastic manifestations and their management
4. Compassionate, supportive approach with recognition of limited treatment options

References:
1. Bitran JD, Ultmann JE, Malignancies of undetermined primary origin. Disease-a-Month 1992;38:216–260.
2. Hainsworth JD, Greco FA, Treatment of patients with cancer of an unknown primary site. Drug therapy. N Engl J Med 1993;329:257–263.

13

HEMATOLOGIC NEOPLASMS

ACUTE MYELOID LEUKEMIA (AML)

CONSULTANT: Peter H. Wiernick, M.D.—Hematologist/Medical Oncologist

Accounts for 80–85% of all cases of acute leukemia in adults over age 20. Is frequently medically induced with radiation or drugs, especially alkylating agents used in treatment of malignancies.

INCIDENCE AND SURVIVAL

	Total	Male	Female
Incidence rate per 100,000/yr	2.3	2.9	1.8
Mortality rate per 100,000/yr	1.7	2.2	1.4
5-year relative survival rate	10.0%	8.4%	12.0%
New cancer cases (est 1994)	7400	3900	3500
Cancer deaths (est 1994)	5100	2800	2300

Trends
Incidence and mortality have decreased slightly over the past two decades. About 80% of young adults and 65% of all patients can achieve complete remission (CR). From 15% to 30% of these CRs will go on to long-term survival with probable cure.

Major risk factors
Ionizing radiation, alkylating chemotherapy drugs, cigarette smoking, occupational exposures (benzene, petroleum refining, etc), myelodysplastic syndromes, aplastic anemia, Fanconi anemia, Bloom's, Kostmann's, Klinefelter's, and Down's syndromes, some viruses.

Pathology (major types)
FAB (French-American-British) classification of AML:

M 0	Minimally differentiated AML
M 1	Myeloid leukemia without maturation
M 2	Myeloid leukemia with maturation
M 3	Promyelocytic leukemia
M 4	Myelomonocytic leukemia
M 5	Monocytic leukemia
M 6	Erythroleukemia
M 7	Megakaryocytic leukemia

Metastatic sites (major)
Liver and spleen.

Associated malignancies
Hodgkin's disease, non-Hodgkin's lymphoma, and plasma cell neoplasm.

Therapy
Combination chemotherapy, bone marrow transplantation, differentiation therapy (all-trans-retinoic acid for promyelocytic leukemia).

Recommendations to patient
Avoid exposure to infection and have it treated promptly when it occurs.

Recommendations to family
Obtain genetic counseling if familial association is involved. Participation in support groups or psychosocial counseling is often helpful to both the patient and the family.

FOLLOW-UP OF THE PATIENT WITH ACUTE MYELOID LEUKEMIA

	1st–3rd Year	Every Year Thereafter (Months)			
	Monthly	3	6	9	12
History					
Complete	X	X	X	X	X
Appetite, weight	X	X	X	X	X
Activity	X	X	X	X	X
Pallor	X	X	X	X	X
Bruising	X	X	X	X	X
Fevers	X	X	X	X	X
Infections	X	X	X	X	X
Lumps	X	X	X	X	X
Bony pain	X	X	X	X	X
Physical					
Complete (yearly)					
Skin	X	X	X	X	X
Lymph nodes	X	X	X	X	X
Chest	X	X	X	X	X
Neurologic	X	X	X	X	X
Fundi	X	X	X	X	X
Tests					
CBC with diff	X	X	X	X	X
Bone marrow (every 3 months if CBC and diff okay)	X				

Comments: After discharge from the hospital following initial chemotherapy, the frequency with which patients treated for acute leukemia need follow-up is dependent on the efficacy of the induction regimen. Those patients in complete remission need frequent observation until the peripheral blood is reconstituted: this usually requires a twice weekly measurement of counts and administration of blood component therapy as needed (packed red blood cells at HCT less than 22–25%; platelets for counts less than 20,000). In the setting of leukopenia, vigilant attention to any signs or symptoms of infection is essential with rehospitalization for any fever higher than 100.6°F.

Once the peripheral blood is reconstituted, the frequency of blood checks can be lengthened to monthly intervals. Since consolidation or intensive therapy is subsequently administered, a return to the pancytopenia state requires a repetition of the initial frequent laboratory measurements and examinations. At the completion of chemotherapy, patients should be seen monthly for the first 3 years. The intervals between appointments for patients in complete bone marrow remission may then be lengthened to 3 months. Repeat marrows are done at the times indicated by the managing hematologist/oncologist.

Failure to enter a remission calls for rehospitalization.

CHRONIC MYELOGENOUS LEUKEMIA (CML)
CONSULTANT: George P. Canellos, M.D.—Hematologist/Medical Oncologist

Accounts for 15% of all patients with leukemia. It was the first major neoplasm characterized by a cytogenetic disorder, the Philadelphia chromosome (Ph 1), which is present in 90–95% of cases. More recently, it was further characterized by the presence of the chimeric *bcr-abl* gene, which is found in some of the cases that are Ph 1 negative; those that have neither are thought to be cases of myelodysplastic syndrome, chronic myelomonocytic leukemia, or related disorders. CML is a clonal myeloproliferative disorder of a pluripotent stem cell with involvement of myeloid, erythroid, megakaryocytic, and occasional B lymphoid cells.

INCIDENCE AND SURVIVAL

	Total	Male	Female
Incidence rate per 100,000/yr	1.3	1.7	1.0
Mortality rate per 100,000/yr	0.8	1.0	0.6
5-year relative survival rate	22.8%	21.3%	24.8%
New cancer cases (est 1994)	4000	2300	1700
Cancer deaths (est 1994)	2400	1300	1100

Trends
Incidence and mortality have decreased over the past two decades.

Major risk factors
Ionizing radiation and cigarette smoking.

Pathology (major types)
Myelocytic progressing to myeloblastic bone marrow as chronic phase progresses to accelerated phase and finally to blast crisis.

Metastatic sites (major)
Liver and spleen.

Associated malignancies
Acute leukemia.

Therapy
Chemotherapy, immunotherapy, and bone marrow transplantation.

Recommendations to patient
Check with family to find HLA-compatible relatives for possible bone marrow transplant in early chronic phase if young enough. Avoid exposure to infection and have it treated promptly when it occurs.

Recommendations to family
Do not expose patient to known infection. In spite of chromosomal translocation, the disease appears to be acquired and not hereditary and does not seem to be familial.

FOLLOW-UP OF THE PATIENT WITH CHRONIC MYELOGENOUS LEUKEMIA

	1st Year (Months)					2nd–5th Year (Months)				Thereafter (Months)
	1	3	6	9	12	3	6	9	12	12
History										
Complete					X				X	X
Appetite, weight	X	X	X	X		X	X	X		
Activity	X	X	X	X		X	X	X		
Pallor	X	X	X	X		X	X	X		
Bruising	X	X	X	X		X	X	X		
Fevers, infections	X	X	X	X		X	X	X		
Bone pain	X	X	X	X		X	X	X		
Enlarged nodes or masses	X	X	X	X		X	X	X		
Physical										
Complete					X				X	X
Skin	X	X	X	X		X	X	X		
Lymph nodes	X	X	X	X		X	X	X		
Chest	X	X	X	X		X	X	X		
Abdomen	X	X	X	X		X	X	X		
Neurologic	X	X	X	X		X	X	X		
Tests										
CBC with diff	X	X	X	X	X	X	X	X	X	X
Chest x-ray	X				X				X	X
Liver function	X		X		X		X		X	X
BUN and creatinine	X		X		X				X	X
Uric acid	X		X		X				X	X

Comments: The major complication of cytotoxic therapy is prolonged pancytopenia. This occurs rarely with busulfan and even more rarely with hydroxyurea and interferon. The chronic phase of CML requires adjustment of dosage according to blood counts, and unless there is a transformation to an accelerated or blastic phase, there is no need for frequent radiographic or chemical testing. CT and MRI scans are not usually needed unless specific symptoms direct their use. Adenopathy, bone lesions, and soft tissue masses are usually signs of blastic transformation. Routine lumbar puncture studies are not required unless clinically indicated. For patients treated with high-dose interferon, there is a need for checking liver function and thyroid function periodically.

ACUTE LYMPHOCYTIC LEUKEMIA (ALL)

CONSULTANT: Thomas P. Duffy, M.D.—Hematologist/Medical Oncologist

Although ALL in children is 75% curable with chemotherapy, long-term disease-free survival is achieved in only 20–30% of adults and primarily in the younger age group.

INCIDENCE AND SURVIVAL

	Total	Male	Female
Incidence rate per 100,000/yr	1.5	1.8	1.3
Mortality rate per 100,000/yr	0.6	0.7	0.5
5-year relative survival rate	51.5%	49.7%	53.8%
New cancer cases (est 1994)	4500	2400	2000
Cancer deaths (est 1994)	2200	1000	1200

Trends

Incidence is stable. Mortality is decreasing as survival rate improves. About 15% of cases are of T-cell phenotype and with recent advances in therapy have about the same prognosis as other immunologic subtypes, although T-cell ALL is associated with a higher incidence of mediastinal masses and CNS involvement.

Major risk factors

Ionizing radiation, genetic factors, occupational exposure (adults), chronic myelocytic leukemia, Down's and Bloom's syndromes, ataxia telangiectasia, HTLV-I virus.

Pathology (major types)

FAB (French-American-British) classification of ALL:

L 1   Small uniform cells with scanty cytoplasm and regular-shaped nuclei
L 2   Large nonuniform cells with irregularly shaped nuclei and prominent nucleoli
L 3   Large uniform cells with regular-shaped nuclei and prominent nucleoli and vacuolization of the cytoplasm

Metastatic sites (major)

Liver and spleen. Sanctuary sites in CNS and testes.

Associated malignancies

Chronic myelocytic leukemia.

Therapy

Combination chemotherapy, bone marrow transplantation, and cranial irradiation.

Recommendations to patient

Avoid exposure to infection and have it treated promptly when it occurs.

Recommendations to family

Obtain genetic counseling if familial association is involved. Participation in support groups or psychosocial counseling is often helpful to both the patient and the family.

FOLLOW-UP OF THE PATIENT WITH ACUTE LYMPHOCYTIC LEUKEMIA

	1st Year (Months)					2nd–5th Year (Months)				Thereafter (Months)
	1	3	6	9	12	3	6	9	12	12
History										
Complete					×				×	×
Appetite, weight	×	×	×	×		×	×	×		
Activity	×	×	×	×		×	×	×		
Pallor	×	×	×	×		×	×	×		
Bruising	×	×	×	×		×	×	×		
Fevers	×	×	×	×		×	×	×		
Infections	×	×	×	×		×	×	×		
Lumps	×	×	×	×		×	×	×		
Bony pain	×	×	×	×		×	×	×		
Physical										
Complete					×				×	×
Skin	×	×	×	×		×	×	×		
Lymph nodes	×	×	×	×		×	×	×		
Chest	×	×	×	×			×			
Neurologic	×	×	×	×			×			
Fundi	×	×	×	×			×			
Tests										
CBC with diff	×	×	×	×	×	×	×	×	×	×
Chest x-ray	×		×		×				×	×
Liver function	×	×	×		×		×		×	×
BUN and creatinine	×		×		×				×	×
Bone marrow			×		×				×	

Comments: The frequency with which patients treated for acute leukemia need follow-up is dependent on the efficacy of the induction regimen. Those patients in complete remission need frequent observation until the peripheral blood is reconstituted: this usually requires a twice weekly measurement of counts and administration of blood component therapy as needed (packed red blood cells at HCT less than 22–25%; platelets for counts less than 20,000). In the setting of leukopenia, vigilant attention to any signs or symptoms of infection is esssential with rehospitalization for any development of fever or chills.

Once the peripheral blood is reconstituted, the frequency of blood checks can be lengthened to monthly intervals. Since consolidation or intensive therapy is subsequently administered, a return to the pancytopenia state requires a repetition of the initial frequent laboratory measurements and examinations. At the completion of chemotherapy the intervals between appointments for patients in complete bone marrow remission may be lengthened to 3 months and then to every 6 months. Repeat marrows are done at the times indicated by the managing hematologist/oncologist.

Failure to enter a remission calls for patient examinations that compensate for the life-threatening cytopenias. The schedule of such visits is determined by the level of blood component support demanded and the needs of the patient.

CHRONIC LYMPHOCYTIC LEUKEMIA (CLL)

CONSULTANT: Kanti Roop Rai, M.D.—Hematologist/Medical Oncologist

Accounts for about one-quarter of all cases of leukemia in the United States. Encompasses a spectrum of monoclonal lymphoproliferative disorders that are characterized by accumulation of large numbers of lymphocytes (95% of the time of B phenotype) in peripheral blood.

INCIDENCE AND SURVIVAL

	Total	Male	Female
Incidence rate per 100,000/yr	6.0	4.1	2.0
Mortality rate per 100,000/yr	1.1	1.7	0.7
5-year relative survival rate	68.1%	66.3%	70.7%
New cancer cases (est 1994)	8000	4900	3100
Cancer deaths (est 1994)	3500	2300	1200
Median survival by Rai stage			
Stage 0	12 years		
Stage I	8 years		
Stage II	6 years		
Stage III	1.5 years		
Stage IV	1.5 years		

Trends

Incidence and mortality have not changed substantially.

Major risk factors

Familial clusters reported, HTLV-I virus.

Pathology (major types)

Lymphocytosis in peripheral blood and bone marrow. Occasional late transformation to Richter syndrome with large lymphocytic (immunoblastic) cells.

Metastatic sites (major)

Enlarged lymph nodes, liver, spleen, lung, and gastrointestinal neoplasms.

Associated malignancies

Hairy cell leukemia, adult T-cell leukemia/lymphoma, prolymphocytic leukemia, and leukemic phase of non-Hodgkin's lymphoma.

Therapy

Chemotherapy.

Recommendations to patient

Avoid exposure to infection and have it treated promptly when it occurs.

Recommendations to patient

Do not expose patient to known infection.

FOLLOW-UP OF THE PATIENT WITH CHRONIC LYMPHOCYTIC LEUKEMIA

1. A patient with CLL who has started the first course of chemotherapy should be seen weekly to monitor chemistries (uric acid, BUN, creatinine, to watch for tumor-lysis syndrome), times 2, then monthly, CBC (to see the pattern of nadiring of absolute neutrophil counts, platelets, lymphocytes, hemoglobin) times 4, then monthly, and physical exam (to see if nodes, spleen, etc, shrink a lot, a bit, or not at all). Chemotherapy dose adjustments for second and subsequent courses are made by taking into consideration the above-noted clinical parameters and during these courses a patient should be seen at a minimum of monthly intervals.

2. Once chemotherapy (or radiation therapy) has been stopped, the patient should be seen at monthly intervals times 3. If there is evidence of stable disease, then see at 3-monthly intervals for 1 year, and if continued stable course, then at 6-monthly intervals indefinitely. If disease is not showing a stable course, frequency of return visit is made monthly (or more often if clinically warranted).

3. At clinic visits, elements of B symptoms of lymphoma are emphasized in the history: weakness, easily fatigued, night sweats, weight loss (without trying), fever (without evidence of overt sepsis), and WHO or Karnofsky performance status score. In the physical exam note size of palpably enlarged nodes, spleen, liver, evidence of gum bleeding, and spontaneous ecchymoses, etc. These findings are considered in relation to findings of preceding visits, whether there is continuing improvement, worsening, or stabilization.

4. Diagnostic imaging: none required routinely.

5. Tumor markers: none required routinely.

6. Blood tests: If anemia develops, direct and indirect Coombs' test should be done. If there is evidence of recurrent bacterial infections, pneumonia, abscess, or frequent urinary tract infections, measurement of serum IgG, IgA, and IgM should be done.

7. CLL patients are at increased risk for developing second malignancies, eg, of gastrointestinal tract, lung, skin, etc. Therefore, during a follow-up visit at 6-month intervals, a re-review of all systems (change in bowel habits, new skin lesions, chest x-rays if considered appropriate) is required.

8. CLL patients terminally develop infections, bleeding, or Richter's transformation, plasmacytoid transformation, or second malignancies. These should be looked for in patients who are not doing well.

HAIRY CELL LEUKEMIA (HCL)

CONSULTANT: Harvey M. Golomb, M.D.—Hematologist/Medical Oncologist

Accounts for about 2% of adult leukemias in the United States. A malignant B-cell lymphoproliferative disease described in the United States since 1958 and formerly called leukemic reticuloendotheliosis.

INCIDENCE AND SURVIVAL

	Total	Male	Female
Incidence rate per 100,000/yr	0.2	0.4	0.1
Mortality rate per 100,000/yr	no data available		
5-year relative survival rate	95%		
New cancer cases (est 1994)	600	480	120
Cancer deaths (est 1994)	no data available		
Median survival duration			
Before chemotherapy and without splenectomy	4.6 years		
Before chemotherapy but with splenectomy	6.9 years		
With current chemotherapy	normal life expectancy		

Trends

With newer therapy, long-term survival and possibly cure should be routine.

Major risk factors

Familial association reported in some cases.

Pathology (major types)

Peripheral blood and bone marrow infiltrated with hairy cells with pale blue to blue-gray agranular cytoplasm with cytoplasmic projections that may be fine and hairlike or broader. Nucleus is sometimes eccentrically placed, may be oval, indented, or even bilobed. Tartrate-resistant acid phosphatase activity is present in 95% of the lymphocytes of patients with HCL.

Metastatic sites (major)

Liver and spleen.

Therapy

Chemotherapy and immunotherapy. Surgery, if needed for splenectomy.

Recommendations to patient

Avoid exposure to infection and have it treated promptly when it occurs.

Recommendations to family

Do not expose patient to known infection. Obtain genetic counseling in cases of familial association.

FOLLOW-UP OF THE PATIENT WITH HAIRY CELL LEUKEMIA

	1st Year (Months)					2nd–5th Year (Months)				Thereafter (Months)
	1	3	6	9	12	3	6	9	12	12
History										
Complete					×				×	×
Appetite	×	×	×	×		×	×	×		
Weight	×	×	×	×		×	×	×		
Activity	×	×	×	×		×	×	×		
Pallor	×	×	×	×		×	×	×		
Bruising	×	×	×	×		×	×	×		
Fevers	×	×	×	×		×	×	×		
Infections	×	×	×	×		×	×	×		
Lumps	×	×	×	×		×	×	×		
Bony pain	×	×	×	×		×	×	×		
Physical										
Complete					×			×		×
Skin	×	×	×	×		×	×	×		
Lymph nodes	×	×	×	×		×	×	×		
Chest	×	×	×	×			×			
Tests										
CBC with diff	×	×	×	×	×	×	×	×	×	×
Chest x-ray					×				×	×
Liver function					×				×	×
BUN and creatinine					×				×	×
Bone marrow	As indicated									

Comments: The course of hairy cell leukemia is usually indolent. If there is an abnormality found on CBC and differential on any visit, and it is of the degree to consider a change or an initiation of therapy, then a bone marrow biopsy should be done (an aspiration alone is insufficient and usually inadequate). Further treatment of HCL is dependent on the level of peripheral blood count and not on the degree of infiltration of the bone marrow by hairy cells. Anemia, leukopenia, thrombocytopenia, and infection are common problems and need to be followed because HCL is controllable and frequently curable with easily tolerable chemotherapy.

PLASMA CELL NEOPLASM
CONSULTANT: Robert A. Kyle, M.D.—Medical Oncologist

The second most common lymphoid malignancy. Monoclonal tumors derived from transformation of a single B-cell lymphocyte or plasma cell.

INCIDENCE AND SURVIVAL

	Total	Male	Female
Incidence rate per 100,000/yr	4.3	5.2	3.6
5-year relative survival rate	27.2%	27.4%	27.0%
New cancer cases (ACS est 1994)	12,700	6,500	6,200
Cancer deaths (ACS est 1994)	9800	5000	4800
5-year relative survival rates by stage			
Stage I	25–40%		
Stage II	15–30%		
Stage III	10–25%		

Trends
Incidence rates have increased over the past two decades, but much of this may be due to improved access to and use of diagnostic techniques by the elderly. Survival has not improved. Incidence and mortality increase with advancing age.

Major risk factors
Ionizing radiation and occupational exposures. Familial history in rare instances.

Pathology (major types)
Plasma cells, plasma blasts.

Metastatic sites (major)
Manifests primarily in bone marrow but can involve any tissue by infiltration. Renal damage may occur.

Associated malignancies
Acute myeloid leukemia and lymphoma.

Therapy
Chemotherapy and radiation.

Recommendations to patient
Seek treatment for infection promptly. Keep well hydrated.

Recommendations to family
Avoid exposing patient to family, friends, or others with known or suspected infections.

FOLLOW-UP OF THE PATIENT WITH PLASMA CELL NEOPLASM

	1st Year (Months)					2nd–5th Year (Months)				Thereafter (Months)
	1	3	6	9	12	3	6	9	12	12
History										
Complete					X				X	X
Appetite, weight	X	X	X	X		X	X	X		
Pallor	X	X	X	X		X	X	X		
Bruising	X	X	X	X		X	X	X		
Fevers	X	X	X	X		X	X	X		
Infections	X	X	X	X		X	X	X		
Lumps	X	X	X	X		X	X	X		
Bony pain	X	X	X	X		X	X	X		
Physical										
Complete					X				X	X
Lymph nodes	X	X	X	X			X			
Chest	X	X	X	X			X			
Abdomen	X	X	X	X		X	X	X		
Tests										
CBC with diff	As needed for chemotherapy									
Chest x-ray	X		X		X				X	X
Serum protein electrophoresis		X	X	X	X		X		X	X
Urine protein electrophoresis*		X	X	X	X				X	X
Skeletal survey			X		X				X	X
Beta-2-microglobulin			X		X				X	
Liver function			X		X		X		X	X
Creatinine, calcium, and uric acid		X	X	X	X	X	X	X	X	X

*24-hour collection if M-protein is present.

Comments: Induction therapy and subsequent treatment of plasma cell neoplasm (multiple myeloma) entails the monthly administration of chemotherapy for 6 to 12 or more months. There is a need for measurement of nadir counts at the midpoint of each cycle in order to adjust the dose of medication to optimal levels. Measurement of renal parameters (creatinine, calcium, and uric acid) is necessary with protein studies at 3-month intervals the first year to document the efficacy of treatment. If remission has been accomplished (decrease of protein spike by 50%, healing of bone lesions, disappearance of proteinuria), an additional 6 months of therapy is administered. At the end of the period, therapy is usually withheld until a rising protein, Bence Jones proteinuria, increased plasmacytosis, and increased beta-2-microglobulin signal reactivation of the disease. Then therapy is begun again in an attempt to induce another response.

HODGKIN'S DISEASE (HD)
CONSULTANTS: Vincent T. DeVita, Jr., M.D.—Medical Oncologist
Dennis Cooper, M.D.—Medical Oncologist

Treatment for HD led the way in showing that tolerable combination chemotherapy could prolong survival and produce cures in advanced cases of what used to be a uniformly fatal disease that afflicts many young people.

INCIDENCE AND SURVIVAL

	Total	Male	Female
Incidence rate per 100,000/yr	2.8	3.3	2.4
Mortality rate per 100,000/yr	0.6	0.8	0.5
5-year relative survival rate	78.1%	75.7%	81.3%
New cancer cases (ACS est 1994)	7900	4400	3500
Cancer deaths (ACS est 1994)	1550	900	650

5- and 10-year survival rates by stage	5-year	10-year
Stage I	90%	90%
Stage II	75–90%	80–90%
Stage III A	65–85%	
Stage III-1		75–90%
Stage III-2		65–80%
Stage III B	50–85%	
Stage III-1		50–80%
Stage III-2		45–70%
Stage IV	40–70%	40–70%

Trends
Incidence decreased slightly over the last two decades while mortality rates internationally have decreased 63% in the past 20 years.

Major risk factors
Epstein-Barr virus and occupational exposure. Associated with higher socioeconomic levels (at least for older age groups).

Pathology (major types)
Sternberg-Reed cell is generally considered pathognomonic. Classical lymphocyte predominant, nodular sclerosing, mixed. Nodular form of lymphocyte predominant now considered a B-cell lymphoma.

Metastatic sites (major)
Neighboring lymph node groups, liver, spleen, and bone marrow.

Associated malignancies
Myeloid leukemia and non-Hodgkin's lymphoma.

Therapy
For newly diagnosed patients, stages I and II, radiation therapy (RT). For stages III and IV, combination chemotherapy (CCT). For patients with massive mediastinal involvement, CCT and RT is indicated. Otherwise, avoid combined therapy because of the risk of an increased incidence of second neoplasms. In patients treated with RT, there is an increased incidence of second solid tumors, particularly lung, breast, and soft tissue sarcomas.

Recommendations to patient
Avoid alcohol use if it triggers pain. Watch for nodes. If treated with RT or chemotherapy that included bleomycin, do not smoke.

FOLLOW-UP OF THE PATIENT WITH HODGKIN'S DISEASE

	1st Year (Months)					2nd–5th Year (Months)			Thereafter (Months)
	1	3	6	9	12	4	8	12	12
History									
Complete					×			×	×
Appetite, weight	×	×	×	×		×	×		
Fever, itching	×	×	×	×		×	×		
Lumps	×	×	×	×		×	×		
Pain, esp alcohol induced	×	×	×	×		×	×		
Night sweats	×	×	×	×		×	×		
Respiratory symptoms	×	×	×	×		×	×		
Physical									
Complete					×			×	×
Lymph nodes	×	×	×	×		×	×		
Chest	×	×	×	×		×	×		
Abdomen	×	×	×	×		×	×		
Liver, spleen	×	×	×	×		×	×		
Oropharynx	×	×	×	×		×	×		
Skin	×	×	×	×		×	×		
Tests									
Chest x-ray		×	×	×	×	×	×	×	×
CBC	×	×	×	×	×	×	×	×	×
Liver function		×			×			×	×
Urine		×			×			×	×
Sedimentation rate		×			×			×	×
CT of chest and abdomen	If initially positive or as indicated								

Comments: Although the complete response rate to initial therapy for advanced Hodgkin's disease is in the range of 80%, and for early stages treated with radiation therapy over 90%, careful follow-up is crucial because 30% of advanced and 20% of early-stage disease will relapse. The earlier the relapse is detected and secondary (rescue) therapy given, the better the chance for second remission and cure. Patients who have no evidence of disease (NED) after careful restaging and who continue NED for 5 years are probably cured, although there are a few relapses up to 8 years. In the rare patient with residual tumor mass on x-ray who is thought to be disease-free, a gallium scan may be useful if the original tumor was gallium avid (positive). For routine follow-up, it has been replaced by the CT scan at 12 months if that was positive at diagnosis.

NON-HODGKIN'S LYMPHOMA (NHL)
Consultants: Vincent T. DeVita, Jr., M.D.—Medical Oncologist
Dennis Cooper, M.D.—Medical Oncologist

Ranked fourth in economic impact of cancers because of large number of patients affected and their relative youth at onset. With combination chemotherapy (CCT), significant prolongation of survival has been achieved. The diffuse large-cell variety is curable by CCT.

INCIDENCE AND SURVIVAL

	Total	Male	Female
Incidence rate per 100,000/yr	13.9	17.1	11.2
Mortality rate per 100,000/yr	6.0	7.5	4.9
5-year relative survival rate	51.7%	49.8%	53.9%
New cancer cases (ACS est 1995)	50,900	29,500	21,400
Cancer deaths (ACS est 1995)	22,700	12,000	10,700

5-year survival rates by stage	I	II	III	IV
Low-grade	80%	80%	70%	60%
Intermediate-grade	80%	50%	50%	50%
High-grade	80%	40%	40%	40%

Trends
Marked increase in incidence and mortality in past two decades especially in men age 20–54, only partially explained by HIV infection. Rates are also increasing in women under age 65 but to a lesser extent.

Major risk factors
Human T-cell leukemia-lymphoma virus, HIV, Epstein-Barr virus (for some forms of high-grade lymphoma), possibly other viruses, genetic immunodeficiency syndromes, organ transplant recipients, patients who received prolonged or high-dose chemotherapy and/or radiation therapy (RT). Pesticides, herbicides, organic solvents, hair coloring products, ionizing radiation (including diagnostic imaging).

Pathology (major types)
Working formulation classifies large multitude of diagnostic entities into low-grade, intermediate-grade, and high-grade.

Metastatic sites (major)
Lymph node groups, liver, spleen, and bone marrow.

Associated malignancies
Myeloid leukemia, lung, brain, kidney, bladder, breast, also melanoma and sarcoma.

Therapy
Low-grade stages I and II without bulky disease are treated with RT to involved fields alone. For bulky stage II and stages III and IV, CCT is the treatment of choice. Interferon is useful. For intermediate- and high-grade stages I and II without bulky disease, CCT is the initial treatment of choice. RT is often added. For bulky stage II and stages III and IV any of several standard drug combinations cures 50% of patients. Surgery is often used as an adjunct to CCT for gastric lymphoma. CNS lymphomas are treated with CCT first, although RT is usually added after remission.

Recommendations to family
Use precautions (latex gloves, etc) when handling body fluids of persons infected or potentially infected with HIV or hepatitis.

FOLLOW-UP OF THE PATIENT WITH NON-HODGKIN'S LYMPHOMA

	1st Year (Months)					2nd–5th Year (Months)			Thereafter (Months)
	1	3	6	9	12	4	8	12	12
History									
Complete					×			×	×
Appetite, weight	×	×	×	×		×	×		
Fever, pain	×	×	×	×		×	×		
Lumps	×	×	×	×		×	×		
Respiratory symptoms	×	×	×	×		×	×		
GI symptoms	×	×	×	×		×	×		
CNS symptoms	×	×	×	×		×	×		
Physical									
Complete					×			×	×
Lymph nodes	×	×	×	×		×	×		
Chest	×	×	×	×		×	×		
Abdomen	×	×	×	×		×	×		
Liver, spleen	×	×	×	×		×	×		
Oropharynx	×	×	×	×		×	×		
Skin	×	×	×	×		×	×		
Neurologic	×	×	×	×		×	×		
Tests									
Chest x-ray		×	×	×	×	×	×	×	×
CBC		×	×	×	×	×	×	×	×
Liver function		×			×			×	×
Urine		×			×			×	×
GI and small-bowel x-ray	As indicated								
CT abdomen and pelvis	If initially positive or as indicated								

*Comments:*Incidence of recurrence is related to histology. Nodular lymphocytic disease is a low-grade lymphoma and may follow an indolent course and go into complete remission, but it almost always recurs. Intermediate- and high-grade lymphomas may have a rapid downhill course with early deterioration and death unless successfully treated with combination chemotherapy. Successfully treated patients have a 50% chance of remaining disease-free and may be cured. Close follow-up is needed in all patients to detect relapse early so that retreatment can be accomplished with curative intent. Relapsed patients whose tumor is still chemotherapy responsive often have a long disease-free survival after high-dose chemotherapy with peripheral blood stem cell or autologous bone marrow support.

CUTANEOUS T-CELL LYMPHOMA

CONSULTANT: Irwin M. Braverman, M.D.—Dermatologist

This designation includes mycosis fungoides and Sézary syndrome. Even the name indicates a new concept and new understanding of this disease as part of the spectrum of malignant lymphomas and the differences between B and T cells and the way that they behave in health and disease.

INCIDENCE AND SURVIVAL

	Total	
Incidence rate per 100,000/yr	0.4	
5-year relative survival rate	73%	
10-year relative survival rate	61%	
5- and 10-year relative survival rates by stage	5-year (%)	10-year (%)
Stage I A	94	89
Stage I B	84	83
Stage II A	82	67
Stage II B	59	31
Stage III	75	48
Stage IV A	20	12
Stage IV B	11	0

Trends
Incidence is rising in the United States: 3.2-fold from 1973 to 1984.

Major risk factors
Unknown.

Pathology (major types)
Infiltration of mononuclear CD-4+ cells in epidermis and upper dermis to eventually form plaques or generalized erythroderma. Later, tumors form and may ulcerate. In Sézary syndrome, these abnormal cells circulate in the peripheral blood.

Metastatic sites (major)
May progress to involve nodes or infiltration of organs including liver, spleen, lung, gastrointestinal tract, and undergo histologic conversion to a high-grade malignancy (large-cell lymphoma).

Associated malignancies
Melanoma. If topical nitrogen mustard or PUVA therapy is used, there is an increased incidence of basal and squamous cell tumors.

Therapy
Radiation, chemotherapy (topical or systemic), immunotherapy, photochemotherapy, and retinoids.

Recommendations to patient
Report recurrent or suspicious skin lesions to physician as soon as noted.

FOLLOW-UP OF THE PATIENT WITH CUTANEOUS T-CELL LYMPHOMA

	1st Year (Months)					2nd–5th Year (Months)			Thereafter (Months)	
	1	3	6	9	12	4	8	12	6	12
History										
Complete					×			×		×
Appetite, weight	×	×	×	×		×	×		×	
Fever	×	×	×	×		×	×		×	
Pruritus	×	×	×	×		×	×		×	
Change in skin lesions	×	×	×	×		×	×		×	
Respiratory symptoms	×	×	×	×		×	×		×	
Other symptoms	×	×	×	×		×	×		×	
Physical										
Complete					×			×		×
Lymph nodes	×	×	×	×		×	×		×	
Chest	×	×	×	×		×	×		×	
Abdomen	×	×	×	×		×	×		×	
Liver, spleen	×	×	×	×		×	×		×	
Skin (most important)	×	×	×	×		×	×		×	
Tests										
CBC	×				×			×		×
Chest x-ray					×	Every 3 years if no symptoms				
Urine		×			×			×		×
CT of abdomen and pelvis	Only when adenopathy or tumors arise									
Liver function		×			×			×		×

Comments: Mycosis fungoides and the Sézary syndrome are neoplasias of malignant T-lymphocytes that usually possess the helper/inducer cell surface phenotype. These lymphomas are low grade and should not be confused with peripheral T-cell lymphomas or adult T-cell leukemia/lymphoma, which may present in the skin. These latter lymphomas are intermediate or high grade, have different staging, and require intensive chemotherapy. The prognosis of cutaneous T-cell lymphomas is based on the extent of disease at presentation (stage). The presence of lymphadenopathy and involvement of peripheral blood and viscera increase in likelihood with worsening cutaneous involvement and define poor prognostic groups. The median survival following diagnosis for all groups is 5–10 years. These disorders are treatable with available topical mechlorethamine (nitrogen mustard), total skin electron beam irradiation, psoralen and ultraviolet A radiation (PUVA), interferons, retinoids, and in advanced cases, systemic chemotherapy (single agent or combination) often combined with treatment to the skin. Patients with stages I and II A disease are potentially curable, but cure in late stages has so far been elusive. About 20% of stages I A, I B, and II A have entered clinical remissions lasting more than 10 years following these therapies. All patients should be followed for a possible relapse and additional therapy, and all patients are candidates for clinical trials evaluating new approaches to treatment.

AIDS-RELATED LYMPHOMA

CONSULTANT: Alexandra M. Levine, M.D.—Medical Oncologist

Non-Hodgkin's lymphoma (NHL) is the second most prevalent malignancy in patients infected with HIV, and its incidence is increasing rapidly. NHL occurs 60–100 times more frequently in AIDS patients than in the general population. It is seen in all groups at risk for AIDS. In contrast, although Hodgkin's disease can occur in the setting of HIV infection, particularly among intravenous drug users, its incidence has not increased and it is not considered an AIDS-defining diagnosis.

Trends

Tends to parallel the incidence of AIDS among homosexual/bisexual men, but increases in incidence with increasing duration of survival with HIV infection. The prolongation of survival with therapy has not yet improved overall mortality rate, although complete remission is expected in approximately 50–60% of treated patients.

Major risk factors

HIV.

Pathology (major types)

Intermediate and high-grade B-cell lymphoma, primarily of the diffuse small noncleaved cell, immunoblastic, and large-cell types.

Metastatic sites (major)

CNS (brain and leptomeninges in 60% of patients throughout the course of the disease and 30% of patients at presentation); gastrointestinal tract (25%), bone marrow (25%), liver (10%), lung, rectum, heart, and literally any other site.

Associated malignancies

Kaposi's sarcoma and perianal squamous cell carcinoma.

Therapy

Chemotherapy; radiation to known CNS involvement.

Recommendations to patient

Be careful not to expose others to your body secretions, which might transmit HIV.

Recommendations to family

Observe universal precautions to protect against transmission of HIV when handling body fluids. Do not expose patient to infection if possible.

FOLLOW-UP OF THE PATIENT WITH AIDS-RELATED LYMPHOMA

	1st Year (Months)												2nd–5th Year (Months)						Thereafter (Months)
	1	2	3	4	5	6	7	8	9	10	11	12	2	4	6	8	10	12	12
History																			
Complete												×						×	×
Pain	×	×	×	×	×	×	×	×	×	×	×	×	×	×	×	×	×		
Appetite, weight	×	×	×	×	×	×	×	×	×	×	×	×	×	×	×	×	×		
Fever	×	×	×	×	×	×	×	×	×	×	×	×	×	×	×	×	×		
Lumps	×	×	×	×	×	×	×	×	×	×	×	×	×	×	×	×	×		
GI symptoms	×	×	×	×	×	×	×	×	×	×	×	×	×	×	×	×	×		
CNS symptoms	×	×	×	×	×	×	×	×	×	×	×	×	×	×	×	×	×		
Respiratory symptoms	×	×	×	×	×	×	×	×	×	×	×	×	×	×	×	×	×		
Physical																			
Complete												×						×	×
Lymph nodes	×	×	×	×	×	×	×	×	×	×	×	×	×	×	×	×	×		
Chest	×	×	×	×	×	×	×	×	×	×	×	×	×	×	×	×	×		
Abdomen	×	×	×	×	×	×	×	×	×	×	×	×	×	×	×	×	×		
Liver, spleen	×	×	×	×	×	×	×	×	×	×	×	×	×	×	×	×	×		
Skin	×	×	×	×	×	×	×	×	×	×	×	×	×	×	×	×	×		
Neurologic	×	×	×	×	×	×	×	×	×	×	×	×	×	×	×	×	×		
Tests																			
Chest x-ray	As indicated											×						×	×
CBC	×	×	×	×	×	×	×	×	×	×	×	×	×	×	×	×	×	×	×
Liver function	×	×	×	×	×	×	×	×	×	×	×	×	×	×	×	×	×	×	×
LDH	×	×	×	×	×	×	×	×	×	×	×	×	×	×	×	×	×	×	×
Urine	As indicated																		
GI x-rays	As indicated																		
CT of abdomen and pelvis			×					×										×	×

Comments: Factors associated with poor prognosis include an AIDS diagnosis prior to the lymphoma; CD-4 cells <200; Karnofsky performance status <70%; stage IV (especially marrow involvement). Systemic chemotherapy is required for these patients with HIV-related lymphoma, despite apparent localization of disease in some. Low-dose chemotherapy may be associated with durable remission in 40–50% of patients. Consolidation radiation therapy to the initial site of bulk disease should be considered and CNS prophylaxis is mandatory. Unfortunately, the appropriate management of patients with primary CNS lymphoma is yet unknown, although studies are attempting to define an effective treatment strategy employing combinations of chemotherapy and cranial radiation.

14

CHILDHOOD CANCERS

CHILDHOOD BRAIN TUMOR (CBT)
CONSULTANT: ROGER J. PACKER, M.D.—Pediatric Neurologist

The most common solid tumor of children, accounting for about 20% of all childhood cancer and increasing in incidence.

INCIDENCE AND SURVIVAL

	Total	Male	Female
Incidence rate per 100,000 children/yr	3.0	3.2	2.7
Mortality rate per 100,000 children/yr	0.8	0.8	0.7
5-year relative survival rate	62.5%		

Survival rates by pathologic tumor type	2-yr (%)	5-yr (%)	10-yr (%)
Infratentorial tumors			
Astrocytoma (low grade)			80
Medulloblastoma (PNET*)		50	
Ependymoma		25–60	
Brain stem glioma	<30		
Supratentorial tumors			
Astrocytoma (low grade)		50–80	
Glioma (low grade)		50–80	
Glioblastoma multiforme	30		
Primitive neuroectodermal tumor		20–40	
Craniopharyngioma			80
Optic tract glioma			80
Pineoblastoma	<50		

*Primitive neuroectodermal tumor.

Trends
Incidence increasing but mortality rate decreasing as survival is increasing.

Major risk factors
Familial cases: neurofibromatosis type I, Li-Fraumeni, Lindau–von Hippel, tuberous sclerosis, Turcot, and ataxia telangiectasia syndromes. Ionizing radiation and some organic chemicals.

Metastatic sites (major)
Medulloblastoma metastasizes most frequently (5–35% of patients) and usually subarachnoid spaces (90%) or bone marrow, lymph nodes, lung, and liver (10%).

Associated malignancies
Other tumors of the Li-Fraumeni syndrome; basal cell carcinoma in nevoid basal cell carcinoma syndrome.

Therapy
Surgery, radiation, and chemotherapy.

Recommendations to family
Obtain genetic counseling if hereditary influence is involved.

FOLLOW-UP OF THE PATIENT WITH CHILDHOOD BRAIN TUMOR

Follow-up is dependent on the histologic type of tumor, its location within the nervous system, and whether the tumor was localized or disseminated at diagnosis. Childhood tumor can be broadly separated into two groupings based on prognosis, rate of growth, and proclivity to disseminate:

Category I: *High risk for early relapse* (starred lesions likely to disseminate). Medulloblastoma,* pineoblastoma,* cortical PNET,* high-grade glioma, ependymoma, germ cell tumor,* pineocytoma, brain stem glioma, and choroid plexus carcinoma.* **Category II:** *Lower risk for early relapse* (late relapse more likely). Cerebellar astrocytoma, other low-grade astrocytoma, craniopharyngioma, and choroid plexus carcinoma.

	1st Year (Months)				2nd–3rd Year (Months)				4th–5th Year (Months)	
	3	6	9	12	6	12	18	24	12	24
CATEGORY I										
Complete history		×		×		×		×	×	×
Focused neurologic history	×	×	×	×	×	×	×	×	×	×
Complete physical (incl height)		×		×		×		×	×	×
Complete neurologic exam	×	×	×	×	×	×	×	×	×	×
MR of head ± contrast	×	×	×	×	×	×	×	×	×	×
MR of spine ± contrast	×[1,*]	×[1]	×[1,*]	×[1]		×[1]		×[1,*]		
Cerebrospinal fluid evaluation	×[*]	×[*]	×[*]	×[*]	×[*]			×[*]		
CBC	Yearly, if received RT or chemotherapy									
EEG	Only as indicated									
T₄, TSH				×[2]		×[2]		×[2]	×[2]	×[2]
Neurocognitive testing		×				×		×		
CATEGORY II										
Complete history		×		×		×		×	×	×
Focused neurologic history	×	×		×		×		×	×	×
Complete physical (incl height)		×		×		×		×	×	×
Complete neurologic exam	×	×		×		×		×	×	×
MR of head ± contrast		×		×		×		×	×	×
MR of spine ± contrast	Only in symptomatic patients									
Cerebrospinal fluid evaluation	Only if positive									
CBC	Only after RT or chemotherapy									
EEG	Only as indicated									
T₄, TSH				×[3]		×[3]		×[3]	×[3]	×[3]
Neurocognitive testing				×[4]			×[4]		×[4]	

×[*] = If positive at diagnosis.
×[1] = For patient likely to disseminate, see above.
×[2] = For those receiving sellar or craniospinal RT
×[3] = In those receiving sellar RT.
×[4] = In those with difficulties.

Comments: With the availability of MR, the majority of patients should be followed by MR with and without contrast. If not available, CT with and without dye can be used. Given the proclivity of some tumors to disseminate the neuroaxis, MR of the spine is part of the follow-up, but should be primarily done in patients with disseminated disease at diagnosis. Given the low rate of extraneural relapse, testing by CXR or other studies is of little yield. Blood counts are primarily needed in patients who have received radiotherapy and/or chemotherapy. Patients should be evaluated for extent of disease immediately following surgery, prior to initiation of further treatment. This includes neuroimaging of the primary tumor site in all patients. Those with tumors that frequently spread through the subarachnoid space require pre- or postoperative MR of the spine and cytologic evaluation. Frequency of follow-up spine and CSF studies is based on initial findings.

In those patients who receive extensive cranial irradiation, sequential neurocognitive and endocrinologic follow-ups are also indicated, as late sequelae are often present. In those receiving craniospinal radiotherapy or sellar radiotherapy, thyroid functions should be obtained yearly. In pre-pubertal children, growth evaluation should be done yearly.

Overall survival has improved for children with some forms of brain tumors, such as medulloblastoma and possibly high-grade gliomas, due to multimodality treatment with surgery, radiotherapy, and chemotherapy. For other tumor types, such as brain stem gliomas, progress has been minimal. Treatment and follow-up are multidisciplinary. Late relapse occurs in both benign and malignant tumors. Anticonvulsants are now infrequently used prophylactically, especially in subtentorial tumors. Even most patients with supratentorial tumors can be safely withdrawn from anticonvulsants.

CHILDHOOD LIVER CANCER (CLC)

CONSULTANT: Edwin C. Douglass, M.D.—Pediatric Oncologist

The tenth most common tumor in children, causing 0.5–2.0% of pediatric tumors. It usually presents as a painless abdominal mass in children. Hepatoblastoma (HB) occurs in children younger than age 5 and hepatocellular carcinoma (HCC) occurs in older children. About 60% of childhood liver tumors are malignant. Of the benign tumors, 60% are hemangiomas or hamartomas.

INCIDENCE AND SURVIVAL

	Total
Incidence rate per 100,000 children/yr (CLC)	0.16
Incidence rate per 100,000 children/yr (HB)	0.09
Incidence rate per 100,000 children/yr (HCC)	0.07
5-year relative survival rate	33%

2-year relative survival rates by group	Hepatoblastoma (%)
Group I	93
Group II	90
Group III	66
Group IV	25
	Hepatocellular carcinoma (%)
Group I/II	50–90
Group III/IV	<10

Major risk factors

Hepatoblastoma: familial cancers. Hepatocellular carcinoma: hepatitis B virus infection, cirrhosis, anabolic steroids (eg, oxymethalone, methyltestosterone, testosterone enanthate, methandienone).

Pathology (major types)

Hepatoblastoma (54%), hepatocellular carcinoma (35%), hepatic sarcomas (11%).

Metastatic sites (major)

Lung and bone.

Associated malignancies

Wilms' tumor and rhabdomyosarcoma.

Associated disorders

Osteopetrosis, hemihypertrophy, neurofibromatosis, lipid storage disease, hereditary tyrosinemia, biliary atresia, de Toni-Fanconi, Beckwith-Wiedemann, ataxia telangiectasia syndromes, and precocious puberty.

Therapy

Surgery, chemotherapy, and radiation.

Recommendations to family

Obtain genetic counseling if hereditary influence is involved, especially familial adenomatous polyposis.

FOLLOW-UP OF THE PATIENT WITH CHILDHOOD LIVER CANCER

	1st–2nd Year (Months)				3rd–5th Year (Months)		Thereafter (Months)
	3	6	9	12	6	12	12
History							
Complete				×		×	×
Appetite, weight	×	×	×		×		
Jaundice, itching	×	×	×		×		
Nausea, vomiting	×	×	×		×		
Abdominal pain	×	×	×		×		
Urine color	×	×	×		×		
Bowel function	×	×	×		×		
Physical							
Complete				×		×	×
Abdominal mass	×	×	×		×		
Liver	×	×	×		×		
Jaundice	×	×	×		×		
Ascites	×	×	×		×		
Tests							
Chest x-ray	×	×	×	×		×	×
CBC	×	×	×	×	×	×	×
Alpha-fetoprotein		×		×	×	×	×
CT or U/S of abdomen	×	×	×	×	×	×	×
CT of chest	Only if alpha-fetoprotein is positive						

Comments: CT scan is the most sensitive way of detecting recurrence of liver tumors. However, ultrasound can be an excellent substitute. HIDA scan can show obstruction and dilatation of the ducts. Alpha-fetoprotein is an extremely sensitive marker for recurrence of hepatoblastoma; any increase should prompt investigation for metastatic sites (CT of chest, CT/MRI of liver).

CHILDHOOD SOFT TISSUE SARCOMA (CSTS)
CONSULTANT: James S. Miser, M.D.—Pediatric Oncologist

Accounts for 6% of all childhood tumors of which half are rhabdomyosarcoma (see discussion of follow-up of rhabdomyosarcoma beginning on page 144). Although adult soft tissue sarcomas are more common, prognosis is better in CSTS, particularly in the younger age groups. Their behavior in adolescents is more like that in adults.

INCIDENCE AND SURVIVAL

	Total	Male	Female
Incidence rate per 100,000 children/yr	0.8	0.9	0.8
Mortality rate per 100,000 children/yr	0.2	0.2	0.2
5-year relative survival rate	69.6%		
New cancer cases (est 1994)	500		

Trends
Incidence is increasing, mortality is decreasing, and survival is increasing.

Major risk factors
Von Recklinghausen's neurofibromatosis, ionizing radiation, familial syndromes, and Li-Fraumeni syndrome.

Pathology (major types)
Fibrosarcoma, neurofibrosarcoma (malignant schwannoma), leiomyosarcoma (LMS), synovial sarcoma (SS), liposarcoma, hemangiopericytoma (HPC), alveolar soft-part sarcoma, malignant fibrous histiocytoma (MFH), epithelioid sarcoma (ES), and angiosarcomas.

Metastatic sites (major)
Lymph nodes (especially SS, ES, MFH, and HPC), lung (all sarcomas—the most frequent site of metastases), bone (especially HPC and ES, otherwise not common), CNS (more common in tumors metastatic to other sites, and MFH, HPC, and those primary in the lungs), and liver (especially LMS of stomach).

Associated malignancies
In the Li-Fraumeni syndrome (breast, glioma, leukemia, adrenocortical carcinoma).

Therapy
Surgery, radiation, and chemotherapy.

Recommendations to family
Obtain genetic counseling in the rare cases where hereditary influence is involved.

FOLLOW-UP OF THE PATIENT WITH CHILDHOOD SOFT TISSUE SARCOMA

	1st Year (Months)					2nd–3rd Year (Months)			4th–5th Year (Months)		Thereafter (Months)
	0	3	6	9	12	4	8	12	6	12	12
History											
Complete	X	X	X	X	X	X	X	X	X	X	X
Pain, mass, abdominal	X	X	X	X	X	X	X	X	X	X	X
Systemic symptoms	X	X	X	X	X	X	X	X	X	X	X
Appetite, growth	X	X	X	X	X	X	X	X	X	X	X
Cardiorespiratory	X	X	X	X	X	X	X	X	X	X	X
CNS	X	X	X	X	X	X	X	X	X	X	X
Distal neurovascular	X	X	X	X	X	X	X	X	X	X	X
Physical											
Complete	X	X	X	X	X	X	X	X	X	X	X
Primary site	X	X	X	X	X	X	X	X	X	X	X
Regional lymph nodes	X	X	X	X	X	X	X	X	X	X	X
Chest	X	X	X	X	X	X	X	X	X	X	X
Abdomen	X	X	X	X	X	X	X	X	X	X	X
Distal neurovascular	X	X	X	X	X	X	X	X	X	X	X
Tests											
Chest x-ray	X	X	X	X	X	X	X	X	X	X	X
CT of chest	X	X	X	X	X	X	X	X	X	X	X
X-ray of primary site	X	Only as indicated									
MRI of primary site	X	X	X		X		X			X	X

MRI performed at diagnosis, prior to surgical extirpation of tumor and follow-up.

CT of primary site is usually used for chest and abdominal primaries.

CT of liver	Only if diagnosis is gastric LMS—f/u as for CT of primary site
Technetium bone scan	f/u scans only if initially positive or if diagnosis is HPC
CT scan of head	Performed if other metastases are present, if diagnosis is HPC, if primary in lungs, or underlying condition is von Recklinghausen's disease— f/u per MRI of primary site
MRI of regional lymph nodes	Performed initially if diagnosis is SS, ES, MFH, or HPC/extremity

CBC	X	f/u as indicated depending on therapy
Renal function	X	f/u as indicated, especially if cisplatin/ifosfamide is used
Liver function	X	f/u as indicated depending on therapy
Audiogram		f/u as indicated, especially if cisplatin is used
Heart function		f/u as indicated, especially if anthracyclines are used

Comments: These tumors, while lumped together, are really heterogenous in presentation, prognosis, and need for follow-up. Several of the tumors should be evaluated in different ways because of patterns of spread that are different. Liver-spleen scans are almost never indicated in children. CTs stage the liver well. Bone scans are only indicated if they are initially positive or the pattern of spread of the tumor is to bone. CT scans of the chest are better generally if done more frequently earlier in the course and less frequently later. Plain chest x-rays are an excellent tool for follow-up and are often all that is needed at a follow-up visit.

NEUROBLASTOMA

CONSULTANTS: Robert P. Castleberry, Jr., M.D.—Pediatric Oncologist
Diane M. Komp, M.D.—Pediatric Oncologist

A tumor of the peripheral nervous system and the most common extracranial solid tumor of childhood, accounting for 8–10% of all childhood cancers. About 85% occur in children under 6 years of age with a median age of 2 years at diagnosis.

INCIDENCE AND SURVIVAL

	Total
Incidence rate per 100,000 children/yr	1.0
5-year relative survival rate	56.5%
New cancer cases (est 1990)	525
5-year relative survival rates by risk group	
Low- or intermediate-risk tumors (40% of cases)	80–95%
High-risk tumors (60% of cases)	<10%

Trends

Patients who are less than 1 year of age at diagnosis generally do better than older children. Elevated levels of serum ferritin, LDH, and neuron-specific enolase (NSE), amplified MYCN oncogene (formerly called N-myc) and DNA index are seen in advanced disease and are poor prognostic signs. Mortality decreasing as survival increases with therapy.

Major risk factors

The tumor originates in the adrenal medulla and/or sympathetic nervous system tissue. There is a genetic predisposition with autosomal dominant pattern of inheritance in some families.

Pathology (major types)

Neuroblastoma, ganglioneuroblastoma, ganglioneuroma. Variable histology. The undifferentiated form has sheets of small round blue cells with scant cytoplasm and little stroma. More differentiated forms have neurofibrillary stroma. About 85% of patients have elevated homovanillic acid (HVA) or vanillymandelic acid (VMA) titers.

Metastatic sites (major)

Bone, bone marrow, lymph nodes, liver, and skin.

Associated malignancies

Pheochromocytoma, brain tumors, acute leukemia, and renal cell carcinoma.

Therapy

Surgery, radiation, chemotherapy, and immunotherapy.

Recommendations to patient

Check to see if eligible to participate in tests of isotretinoin (13-cis-retinoic acid) differentiation therapy.

Recommendations to family

Obtain genetic counseling if familial involvement is suspected.

FOLLOW-UP OF THE PATIENT WITH NEUROBLASTOMA

	1st Year (Months)					2nd–5th Year (Months)				Thereafter (Months)
	1	3	6	9	12	3	6	9	12	12
History										
Complete					×				×	×
Appetite, weight	×	×	×	×		×	×	×		
Activity	×	×	×	×		×	×	×		
Pallor	×	×	×	×		×	×	×		
Bruising	×	×	×	×		×	×	×		
Fevers	×	×	×	×		×	×	×		
Infections	×	×	×	×		×	×	×		
Lumps	×	×	×	×		×	×	×		
Bony pain	×	×	×	×		×	×	×		
Behavioral changes	×		×			×				
Physical										
Complete					×				×	×
Blood pressure	×	×	×	×		×	×	×		
Growth parameters	×	×	×	×			×			
Developmental		×	×				×			
Tests										
CBC with diff	×	×	×	×	×	×	×	×	×	×
Catecholamines (urine)	×	×	×	×	×		×		×	
Chest x-ray	×		×		×				×	
CT of primary or U/S	×		×		×		×		×	
Bone scan, x-rays	if metastases present at diagnosis									
Echocardiogram			×		×					
Audiogram		×	×		×				×	
Liver function	×	×	×		×		×		×	
BUN and creatinine	×		×		×					

Comments: Follow-up of childhood cancer involves complex developmental and psychosocial issues in addition to monitoring for recurrence of malignancy. All childhood cancers should be followed by specially trained pediatric oncologists at a tertiary care center where coordination with pediatric surgery and neurosurgery, neurology, endocrinology, developmental physiology, radiotherapy, as well as the special needs that long-term pediatric cancer survivors have in the sphere of social services, physical therapy, and genetic counseling, are easily accessible. The above guidelines presume an abdominal/pelvic primary that is not completely resected at the time of diagnosis. Individual cases may need closer or slightly less frequent follow-up depending on the initial presentation and the modalities of treatment given (surgery, chemotherapy, and/or radiation). Patients with the best prognosis are those who were under the age of 1 year with completely resected primary tumors and no local lymph node or distant metastatic disease.

RHABDOMYOSARCOMA

CONSULTANT: R. Beverly Raney, Jr., M.D.—Pediatric Oncologist

This is the most common soft tissue sarcoma of children and accounts for 5–8% of all childhood cancers. It is frequently grouped with the childhood soft tissue sarcomas of which it comprises approximately half. It is treated here as a separate entity to include all tumors that arise from tissue that looks like muscle histologically and histochemically (with desmin positivity).

INCIDENCE AND SURVIVAL

	Total	Male	Female
Incidence rate per 100,000 children/yr	0.8	0.5	0.3
Mortality rate per 100,000 children/yr	0.2	0.1	0.1
5-year relative survival rate	60%		
5-year relative survival if mets at diagnosis	<30%		
New cancer cases (est 1994)	250–300		
5-year relative survival rates by IRS* grouping			
Group I	90%		
Group II	80%		
Group III	65%		
Group IV	27%		

Note: *IRS = Intergroup Rhabdomyosarcoma Study. The IRS now uses a modified TNM staging system, but no reliable 5-year data are available yet by that system.

Trends

Incidence is stable, mortality is decreasing, and survival is increasing.

Major risk factors

Von Recklinghausen's neurofibromatosis, ionizing radiation, familial syndromes. Li-Fraumeni, Rubinstein-Taybi, and Roberts' syndromes.

Pathology (major types)

Embryonal, botryoid, alveolar, undifferentiated sarcoma.

Metastatic sites (major)

Lymph nodes, lung, bone marrow, bone, CNS, heart, liver, and breast.

Associated malignancies

Maternal breast in the Li-Fraumeni syndrome.

Therapy

Surgery, radiation, and chemotherapy.

Recommendations to family

Obtain genetic counseling if hereditary influence is involved.

FOLLOW-UP OF THE PATIENT WITH RHABDOMYOSARCOMA

	1st–2nd Year (Months)				3rd Year (Months)			4th–5th Year (Months)		Thereafter (Months)
	3	6	9	12	4	8	12	6	12	12
History										
Complete				X			X		X	X
Appetite, weight	X	X	X		X	X		X		
Pain	X	X	X		X	X		X		
Mass	X	X	X		X	X		X		
Respiratory	X	X	X		X	X		X		
CNS	X	X			X	X		X		
Distal neurovascular	X	X	X		X	X		X		
Physical										
Complete				X			X		X	X
Primary site	X	X	X		X	X		X		
Chest	X	X	X		X	X		X		
Abdomen	X	X	X		X	X		X		
Lymph nodes	X	X	X		X	X		X		
Distal neurovascular	X	X	X		X	X		X		
Tests										
Chest x-ray	X	X	X		X	X		X		X
Chest CT				X			X		X	
CT/MRI of primary site*				X			X		X	
Bone scan				X			X		X	
CBC		X		X			X		X	X
Liver and renal function		X		X			X		X	X
Liver-spleen scan	As indicated									
Additional specific	As indicated									

*Because of their heterogeneous nature, rhabdomyosarcomas, like other soft tissue sarcomas, often require a more customized follow-up approach, reflecting differing patterns of metastasis. For example, tumors in the head and neck are best followed by MRI (preferred) or CT; plain radiographs are of little use due to their poor resolution.

Comments: Primary soft tissue tumors, while rare, affect virtually any site in individuals of all ages. Because of their infrequent nature, these neoplasms are often misdiagnosed, confused with other benign disease, or overlooked. Limb-sparing tumor resections are often feasible, following accurate diagnostic biopsy (needle, or open) and staging. Like primary bone and cartilage tumors, these lesions often benefit from combined surgical, chemotherapeutic, and irradiation approaches. These malignancies tend to metastasize to lung and bone. Unlike primary osseous tumors, plain x-rays are often unrewarding, but the use of CT or MRI scans, angiography, and other selected diagnostic imaging approaches offers excellent resolution of local disease. Close follow-up is important, since aggressive surgical treatment of lung metastases combined with chemotherapy has been associated with substantial long-term survival.

WILMS' TUMOR

CONSULTANTS: *Giulio J. D'Angio, M.D.—Pediatric Radiation Oncologist*
Phillip M. Devlin, M.D.—Radiation Oncologist

Wilms' tumor (WT) is the most common primary malignant renal tumor of the 1–16-year-old age group with an annual incidence of seven per million. There is an equal gender distribution and a mean age of 3 years. Sometimes it is associated with overgrowth syndromes, ie, the Beckwith-Wiedemann syndrome and hemihypertrophy. Ambiguous genitalia or sporadic aniridia, whether or not part of the WAGR (WT, aniridia, genital malformations, mental retardation) syndrome, are also associated conditions. Nephrogenic rests are precursor lesions. Deletions at two loci on the short arm of chromosome 11 (11p13 and 11p15) underlie these findings, but not in familial cases, suggesting one or more other genes are implicated. Siblings of affected patients are at 40 times the normal risk. A mass, often discovered on bathing, is the most common presenting sign.

Work-up is aimed at identifying the tumor as intrarenal and establishing whether there is (1) a functioning contralateral kidney, (2) a thrombus in the renal vein, inferior vena cava, or the right atrium, and (3) metastatic disease (principally in the lungs).

Ninety-two percent of childhood renal tumors are WT (favorable histology [FH]: 87%; anaplastic [Ana]: 6%). Clear cell sarcoma (3%), rhabdoid tumor (<2%), mesoblastic nephroma (<2%), and renal cell carcinoma (<1%) comprise the remainder.

Staging: I = tumor localized to the kidney and completely excised; II = regional extracapsular invasion totally excised, local spillage, and/or tumor thrombus may be present; III = residual regional disease, positive abdominal lymph nodes, and/or massive spillage; IV = distant metastases usually to the lungs or the liver; V = bilateral renal involvement at diagnosis.

Most patients in North America receive postoperative therapy according to the National Wilms' Tumor Study (NWTS). Preoperative chemotherapy is also used, mostly in European centers. Vincristine and dactinomycin form the mainstay of adjuvant therapy with doxorubicin and radiation therapy being reserved for locally advanced and metastatic disease.

The four year overall survival in the fourth NWTS for patients with Stage I Ana and FH tumors of all stages is 95%. Children with higher-stage Ana or other malignant tumors remain at higher risk. There is a 50% overall retrieval rate for relapsed patients.

One in a thousand young adults is a long-term survivor of childhood cancer. Surveillance for iatrogenic complications through adulthood, guided by the type of therapy, is essential; eg, second malignant neoplasms, mostly in irradiated tissues, are seen in 1-2% of NWTS long-term survivors.

FOLLOW-UP OF THE PATIENT WITH WILMS' TUMOR

Physical Examination

Vital signs, abdomen for masses,
the thyroid if lungs were irradiated,
growth pattern, signs of chemotherapy
or radiation toxicity

Frequency

Every 3 months × 5, then every 6 months × 2,
yearly × 3, then prn.

Laboratory tests

CBC and differential
Urinalysis
Creatinine
Liver function

Weekly until normal; then as clinically indicated.
As clinically indicated.
Every 6 months × 2 years, then yearly.
Every 6 months × 2 years, then as clinically indicated.

Radiographs

Chest   Stages I, II, III

Lung metastases at diagnosis

Irradiated bones
screening for second malignancy
Brain and liver scans
Nephroblastomatosis in one or both kidneys

3 months, then every 3 months × 5,
every 6 months × 3, then yearly × 2.
Every 6 weeks until there has been a complete
response in the lung for 9 months, then as above.
x-ray yearly until full growth attained,
then every 5 years.
As clinically indicated.
Abdominal ultrasound (U/S) every 3 months for 5 years
or until 7 years of age.

Screening of Patients with Increased Risk for Wilms' Tumor

Sporadic aniridia, hemihypertrophy,
ambiguous genitalia, Beckwith-Wiedemann, or
WAGR syndrome

U/S every 3 months until 5 years of age, then yearly
until fully grown. Caretakers should be taught
abdominal palpation for frequent (biweekly to
monthly) examination at home.

CHILDHOOD ACUTE MYELOGENOUS LEUKEMIA (cAML)
CONSULTANT: HOWARD J. WEINSTEIN, M.D.—Pediatric Oncologist

Accounts for 15–20% of all pediatric leukemias. When cAML occurs in the first year of life, it is usually of the M 4 and M 5 types.

INCIDENCE AND SURVIVAL

	Total	Male	Female
Incidence rate per 100,000 children/yr (0–14 yr)	0.8	0.9	0.8
Incidence rate per 100,000 children/yr (0–19 yr)	0.7	0.8	0.6
Mortality rate per 100,000 children/yr	0.2	0.3	0.1
5-year relative survival rate	31.6%		
New leukemia cases (est 1994)	400	200	200
Leukemia deaths (est 1994)	280	140	140
Complete remission rate (CR)	75–85%		

Trends
Incidence increasing but this is likely due to improved leukemic diagnosis and prevention of childhood deaths from infectious causes. Mortality rate decreasing as survival is increasing due to improved therapy.

Major risk factors
Ionizing radiation. Some anticancer chemotherapy drugs. Familial leukemia, Down's, Kostmann's, Bloom's, and Klinefelter's syndromes. Fanconi and Diamond-Blackfan anemia. Aplastic anemia, myelodysplastic syndromes, and benzene exposure.

Pathology (major types)
FAB (French-American-British) classification of AML:

M 0	Minimally differentiated AML
M 1	Myeloid leukemia without maturation
M 2	Myeloid leukemia with maturation
M 3	Promyelocytic leukemia
M 4	Myelomonocytic leukemia
M 5	Monocytic leukemia
M 6	Erythroleukemia
M 7	Megakaryocytic leukemia

Metastatic sites (major)
Skin, chloromas (myeloblastomas), CNS, and gums.

Therapy
Chemotherapy. Allogeneic bone marrow transplantation from a matched sibling donor in first remission. All transretinoic acid for acute promyelocytic leukemia with chemotherapy is being compared to chemotherapy alone.

Recommendations to family
Obtain genetic counseling if hereditary influence is involved.

FOLLOW-UP OF THE PATIENT WITH CHILDHOOD ACUTE MYELOGENOUS LEUKEMIA

	At time of diagnosis	1st Year (Months)					2nd–5th Year (Months)				Thereafter (Months)
		1	3	6	9	12	3	6	9	12	12
History											
Complete	X				X				X		X
Appetite, weight	X		X	X	X	X	X	X	X		
Activity	X		X	X	X	X	X	X	X		
Pallor and bruising	X		X	X	X	X	X	X	X		
Fevers	X		X	X	X	X	X	X	X		
Infections	X		X	X	X	X	X	X	X		
Lumps	X		X	X	X	X	X	X	X		
Bony pain	X		X	X	X	X	X	X	X		
Behavioral changes	X		X		X				X		
Physical											
Complete	X				X				X		X
Skin and lymph nodes	X		X	X	X	X	X	X	X		
Chest	X		X	X	X	X		X			
Neurologic	X		X	X	X	X		X			
Fundi	X		X	X	X	X	X	X	X		
Abdomen	X		X	X	X	X	X	X	X		
Growth parameters	X		X	X	X	X		X			
Developmental	X		X	X				X			
Testes	X		X	X	X	X	X	X	X		
Tests											
CBC with diff	X	X	X	X	X	X	X	X	X	X	X
Chest x-ray	X	X									
Liver function	X	X		X		X				X	
BUN and creatinine	X	X		X		X				X	
Bone marrow aspirate	X	X	X	X	X	X					
Spinal tap (cytocentrifuge)	X										
Endocrine	X				X				X		X

Comments: Follow-up of childhood cancer survivors involves complex developmental and psychosocial issues in addition to monitoring for recurrence of malignancy. All survivors of childhood cancers should be followed by specially trained pediatric oncologists at a tertiary care center where coordination with pediatric surgery and neurosurgery, neurology, endocrinology, developmental physiology, radiotherapy, as well as the special needs that long-term pediatric cancer survivors have in the spheres of social services, physical therapy, and genetic counseling, are easily accessible. All children with AML should have a bone marrow aspiration examination prior to going off of therapy. The role of more frequent bone marrow examinations during therapy or within the first 2 years after diagnosis is controversial.

CHILDHOOD ACUTE LYMPHOBLASTIC LEUKEMIA (cALL)
CONSULTANTS: David G. Poplack, M.D.—Pediatric Oncologist
G. Peter Beardsley, M.D.—Pediatric Oncologist/Hematologist

The most common malignancy of children, accounting for almost one-third of all cases of childhood cancer and three-fourths of childhood leukemia. Only 40 years ago, this disease was 100% fatal, and usually in 2–3 months. Now, more than 60% of children treated are disease-free at 5 years and most of them are cured—a remarkable success story, but still room for substantial improvement. The lessons learned in treating cALL have helped in treating other neoplasms.

INCIDENCE AND SURVIVAL

	Total	Male	Female
Incidence rate per 100,000 children/yr (0–14 yr)	3.3	3.7	3.0
Incidence rate per 100,000 children/yr (0–19 yr)	2.8	3.2	2.4
Mortality rate per 100,000 children/yr	0.6	0.7	0.5
5-year relative survival rate	69.5%		
New leukemia cases (est 1994)	2,000		
Leukemia deaths (est 1994)	600		
Complete remission rate (CR)	90–98%		

Trends
Incidence increasing slightly; mortality rate decreasing as survival is greatly increased due to improved therapy. Mortality reduced by 90% in the past two decades.

Prognostic factors/Risk group assignment
Certain clinical and laboratory characteristics/findings evident at diagnosis have prognostic importance. Patient age, the initial WBC, immunophenotype, karyotype, cytogenetic findings, and DNA index are among the most important. These factors are used to define risk groups (eg, high risk, average risk, low risk) based on the projected likelihood of relapse. Therapy is tailored according to risk group.

Pathology (major types)

FAB (FRENCH-AMERICAN-BRITISH) CLASSIFICATION OF ALL

	Cell	Cytoplasm	Nucleoli	Basophilia	Incidence
L 1	small	scant	inconspicuous	slight	85%
L 2	large	abundant	prominent	variable	14%
L 3	large	variable	prominent	deep	1%

Metastatic sites (major)
Sanctuary sites in CNS and testes primarily; also liver, spleen, and kidneys.

Therapy
Given according to treatment protocols with approaches specific for risk groups. Chemotherapy for systemic disease, intrathecal CT with or without cranial radiation as CNS preventive therapy.

Recommendations to family
Treatment should be processed at a children's cancer center. Watch for growth impairment. If CNS radiation was given, watch for intellectual impairment that may require educational assistance.

FOLLOW-UP OF THE PATIENT WITH CHILDHOOD ACUTE LYMPHOBLASTIC LEUKEMIA

	1st Year (Months)					2nd–5th Year (Months)				Thereafter (Months)
	1	3	6	9	12	3	6	9	12	12
History										
Complete					X				X	X
Appetite, (weight)	X	X	X	X		X	X	X		
Activity	X	X	X	X		X	X	X		
Behavioral changes	X	X	X	X		X	X	X		
Pallor, bruising	X	X	X	X		X	X	X		
Fevers	X	X	X	X		X	X	X		
Infections	X	X	X	X		X	X	X		
Lumps	X	X	X	X		X	X	X		
Bony pain	X	X	X	X		X	X	X		
Physical										
Complete					X				X	X
Growth parameters	X	X	X	X			X			
Developmental	X	X	X	X			X			
Skin	X	X	X	X		X	X	X		
Lymph nodes	X	X	X	X		X	X	X		
Chest	X	X	X	X		X	X	X		
Abdomen	X	X	X	X		X	X	X		
Neurologic	X	X	X	X			X			
Testes	X	X	X	X		X	X	X		
Fundi	X	X	X	X		X	X	X		
Tests										
CBC with diff	X	X	X	X	X	X	X	X	X	X
Chest x-ray	X		X		X				X	
Liver function	X		X		X		X		X	
BUN and creatinine	X		X		X				X	X
Endocrine		X			X				X	X

Comments: Follow-up of long-term survivors of childhood cancer involves complex developmental and psychosocial issues in addition to monitoring for recurrence of malignancy. All childhood cancers should be followed by specially trained pediatric oncologists at a tertiary care center where coordination with pediatric surgery and neurosurgery, neurology, endocrinology, development physiology, radiotherapy, as well as the special needs that long-term pediatric cancer survivors have in the sphere of social services, physical therapy, and genetic counseling, are easily accessible. All children with ALL should have a bone marrow aspiration and cerebrospinal fluid examination prior to therapy termination. Bilateral testicular biopsies are required by some protocols. The above suggested guidelines are for *low-risk* ALL. Children in higher-risk categories may require more frequent follow-up. Patients who have experienced a CNS relapse may need more follow-up evaluation of CSF.

CHILDHOOD HODGKIN'S DISEASE (CHD)

CONSULTANTS: Sarah S. Donaldson, M.D.—Radiation Oncologist
Michael P. Link, M.D.—Pediatric Oncologist

A malignant disease of lymph nodes characterized by the presence of multinucleated Reed-Sternberg cells. Rare before the age of 5 years, it has a bimodal age peak, the first in adolescents and young adults and the later peak in elderly individuals.

INCIDENCE AND SURVIVAL

Incidence rate per 100,000 children/yr	Caucasian males	Caucasian females
0–4 yr	0.06	0.07
5–9 yr	0.68	0.25
10–14 yr	1.37	1.67
15–19 yr	3.67	4.18

5-year relative survival rates by stage	Event-free survival (%)	Overall survival (%)
Limited stage, I–II, favorable	85–98	90–100
Advanced stage, III–IV, unfavorable	63–90	72–92

Trends

Incidence unchanged but mortality markedly decreasing. The few deaths today from CHD are usually confined to stage IV unfavorable patients and those who develop a secondary (therapy associated) neoplasm.

Major risk factors

Immunodeficiency syndromes, both acquired (HIV) and hereditary (ataxia telangiectasia syndrome). Epstein-Barr virus infection. Prior history of infectious mononucleosis. Higher family socioeconomic status.

Pathology (major types)

Reed-Sternberg cell is generally considered pathognomonic. Nodular sclerosing and mixed cellularity account for majority; lymphocyte depleted and lymphocyte predominant are rare. Spread is by lymphatic routes (early stage) and hematogenous spread (late stage) to neighboring lymph node groups, liver, spleen, bone marrow, lung, pleura, pericardium, and bone.

Therapy

Combination chemotherapy and radiation for the majority of patients. Radiation therapy alone for select early-stage presentations in fully grown children.

Recommendations to family

Obtain genetic counseling if familial association involved. Late second malignancies occur; acute myeloid leukemia, and its precursor, a pan-myelocytic myelodysplastic syndrome, are seen in patients who received alkylating agent–based chemotherapy. Secondary solid tumors occur 10 or more years following radiation therapy and chemotherapy. Most common solid tumors are lung, gastric, melanoma, bone, and connective tissue tumors. Breast cancer and thyroid cancer are also seen. Children with Hodgkin's disease should be referred to a pediatric cancer center for consultation, treatment, and follow-up.

FOLLOW-UP OF THE PATIENT WITH CHILDHOOD HODGKIN'S DISEASE

	First Year (Months)						2nd Year (Months)				3rd-5th Year (Months)			Thereafter (Months)
	2	4	6	8	10	12	3	6	9	12	4	8	12	12
History														
Complete						×				×			×	×
Appetite, weight	×	×	×	×	×		×	×	×		×	×		
Fever	×	×	×	×	×		×	×	×		×	×		
Lumps	×	×	×	×	×		×	×	×		×	×		
Night sweats	×	×	×	×	×		×	×	×		×	×		
Respiratory symptoms	×	×	×	×	×		×	×	×		×	×		
Physical														
Complete						×				×			×	×
Lymph nodes	×	×	×	×	×		×	×	×		×	×		
Abdomen	×	×	×	×	×		×	×	×		×	×		
Chest	×	×	×	×	×		×	×	×		×	×		
Liver, spleen	×	×	×	×	×		×	×	×		×	×		
Skin	×	×	×	×	×		×	×	×		×	×		
Oropharynx	×	×	×	×	×		×	×	×		×	×		
Tests														
Chest x-ray	×	×	×	×	×	×	×	×	×	×	×	×	×	×
CBC	×	×	×	×	×	×	×	×	×	×	×	×	×	×
Alk phos, LDH	×	×	×	×	×	×	×	×	×	×	×	×	×	×
Sedimentation rate		×				×				×			×	×

Comments: Although the complete response rate to initial therapy in Hodgkin's disease is in the range of 90–99%, careful follow-up is crucial because 10–15% of patients relapse. The earlier the relapse is detected and secondary (rescue) therapy is given, the better the chance for second remission and cure. Patients who have no evidence of disease (NED) after careful restaging, and who continue NED for 5 years, are probably cured, but need to be carefully followed for possible late effects of therapy. In the rare patient with residual tumor mass on x-ray who is thought to be disease-free, close follow-up with laboratory and radiographic evaluation is sufficient, with no intervention needed unless the mass enlarges. All patients with suspected relapse must be biopsied to confirm relapse versus rebound hyperplasia versus a new malignancy.

CHILDHOOD NON-HODGKIN'S LYMPHOMA (CNHL)

CONSULTANTS: Ian T. Magrath, M.D.—Pediatric Oncologist
Aziza T. Shad, M.D.—Pediatric Oncologist

Accounts for 7–10% of childhood malignancies.

INCIDENCE AND SURVIVAL

	Total	Male	Female
Incidence rate per 100,000 children/yr <19 years	1.8	2.5	1.1
Mortality rate per 100,000 children/yr < 19 years	0.5	0.8	0.16
5-year relative survival rate	71%		
New cancer cases (est 1994) < 19 years	405	225	180
5-year relative survival rates by stage			
Stage I	>90%		
Stages II and III	80–90%		
Stage IV	70–80%		

Trends

Incidence increasing significantly, but mortality rate decreasing as survival is greatly increasing due to improved dose-intensive therapy.

Major risk factors

Inherited and acquired immunodeficiencies, eg, Wiskott-Aldrich syndrome, X-linked lymphoproliferative syndrome (XLP), and HIV.

Pathology (major types)

Small noncleaved cell lymphoma (33–50%), lymphoblastic lymphomas (33%), immunoblastic and anaplastic large cell (Ki–1 positive) lymphomas (15–30%).

Metastatic sites (major)

Gastrointestinal tract, mediastinum, pleura, lymph node, CNS, nasopharynx, breast, testes, bone, skin, liver, and spleen (rare).

Therapy

Primary treatment of choice is chemotherapy. Role of radiation is minor. Role of surgery is confined to diagnosis and emergencies.

Recommendations to patient

Lymphadenopathy that is significant and is increasing or not responding to antibiotics should be biopsied.

Recommendations to family

Genetic counseling if there is an inherited immunodeficiency syndrome in the family (eg, Wiskott-Aldrich syndrome, or X-linked lymphoproliferative syndrome).

FOLLOW-UP OF THE PATIENT WITH CHILDHOOD NON-HODGKIN'S LYMPHOMA

	1st Year (Months)					2nd–5th Year (Months)		Thereafter (Months)
	1	3	6	9	12	6	12	12
History								
Complete	X	X	X	X	X	X	X	X
Appetite, weight	X	X	X	X	X	X	X	X
Fever, pain	X	X	X	X	X	X	X	X
Lumps	X	X	X	X	X	X	X	X
Respiratory symptoms	X	X	X	X	X	X	X	X
GI symptoms	X	X	X	X	X	X	X	X
CNS symptoms	X	X	X	X	X	X	X	X
Physical								
Complete	X	X	X	X	X	X	X	X
Lymph nodes	X	X	X	X	X	X	X	X
Chest including heart	X	X	X	X	X	X	X	X
Abdomen	X	X	X	X	X	X	X	X
Liver, spleen	X	X	X	X	X	X	X	X
Oropharynx	X	X	X	X	X	X	X	X
Skin	X	X	X	X	X	X	X	X
Neurologic	X	X	X	X	X	X	X	X
Testes	X	X	X	X	X	X	X	X
Tests								
Chest x-ray	X	X	X	X	X			
CBC	X	X	X	X	X		X	X
Liver function	X	X	X	X	X			
Urine	X	X	X	X	X			
CT of abdomen, pelvis, and chest*					X			
Gallium scan		X	X	X	X			
Bone marrow and CSF	At first f/u after therapy is completed							

*If abnormal at presentation, obtain every 3 months for first year only. Patients with lymphoblastic lymphoma need scans every 3 months for 2 years if abnormal at presentation.

Comments: All pediatric NHL are of high-grade variety and need to be treated with aggressive, dose-intensive, combination chemotherapy regimens. They tend to respond to a wide range of chemotherapeutic agents, partly because of their high growth fraction. Response tends to correlate with histology and immunophenotype. Using the most effective regimens available today, 90% or more of the patients can be expected to achieve complete remission, while the cure rate (ie, no relapse beyond 1 year for the small noncleaved cell lymphomas) is almost 100% in patients with limited disease and 60–90% in patients with extensive disease. Close follow-up, especially for the first year, is essential. Patients with recurrent disease after modern, intensive chemotherapy have a very low chance of survival if retreated with conventional chemotherapy. Such candidates should be considered candidates for massive chemotherapy with or without bone marrow transplantation and/or peripheral stem cell infusions, or for experimental therapy.

15

PREVENTION

fter an individual is diagnosed with a malignancy, the family frequently becomes acutely
aware of the dangers of cancer, which is the second most common cause of death at the
present time in the United States and is expected to become the single most common cause
of death in the next century. Accordingly, the physician can expect to be consulted to advise on
methods to prevent the development of cancer and to detect it as early as possible in what is
hopefully a curative stage. These are two separate endeavors. Here we will attempt to briefly
summarize the highlights of present concepts of prevention.

Cancer begins with the transformation of a normal cell into a malignant cell, which then
reproduces and develops into a clone of cancer cells, which, when big enough to be detected, is
called a malignant tumor. It is not entirely clear how this process occurs in all cases, but it is thought
to occur in stages and over a period of time. It is strongly influenced by genetic factors that are now
being studied and have added to our knowledge of the role of heredity in carcinogenesis. In the
situation of nongenetic predisposition, it is thought that there are three stages in the development of
a cancer: (1) initiation, (2) promotion, and (3) progression. This concept is based to a large extent on
studies of skin cancer development in mice.

Initiation is a rapid and irreversible process caused by exposure to a carcinogen, frequently a
chemical or radiation, that interferes with the normal processes of a cell and starts it on the path to
malignancy. However, in the absence of a promoter, a malignant tumor never develops. Promotion is
a more prolonged process consequent to continuous or repeated exposure to a substance or agent,
which in itself is not carcinogenic or capable of initiating a malignant change, but once the initiator
has started the process, the promoter causes the premalignant cell to become fully malignant. This
cycle has sometimes been called the "two-hit theory." Finally, progression leads to the reproduction
of the malignant cell and its invasion into normal tissues and eventually to metastasis. Prevention
involves avoidance of exposure to the initiator when possible, and even more so to the promoter,
since promotion is a much longer process and allows a better chance to avoid the full development
of the malignancy. Figure 15-1 diagrams the development of metastatic cancer.

FIGURE 15-1.
The development of a metastatic cancer.

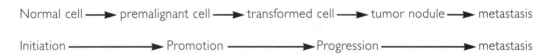

The work of Isaiah J. Fidler and others has shown that the pathway from tumor nodule to
metastasis is far more complex than we had imagined, and provides additional opportunities for
interruption and abortion of metastasis development, which is discussed in a separate chapter. Here
we will discuss what we know or think we know about prevention.

First, it is important to understand the basis for the statements that are made in support of the
evidence, since not all of it is hard scientific fact that is reproducible in the laboratory, for most of it
is not laboratory research but epidemiological observations, clinical trials, cohort or case-control
studies, and even best opinions of experts based on anecdotal observations and clinical experience.

The National Cancer Institute (NCI) has released through its Physician's Data Query (PDQ) a
group of suggestions for prevention of a few of the more common kinds of cancer. They categorize
the various levels of evidence that support a given statement. The strongest evidence would be that
obtained from a well-designed and well-conducted randomized controlled trial with cancer-specific
mortality as the endpoint. It is, however, not always practical or ethical to conduct such a trial to
address every question surrounding the field of cancer prevention. As in many other aspects of

medicine, practice must be based on information that falls short of a randomized trial. For each summary of evidence statement, the associated levels of evidence are listed. In order of strength of evidence, the six levels are as follows:

1. Evidence obtained from at least one randomized controlled trial with:
   (a) a cancer mortality endpoint
   (b) a cancer incidence endpoint
   (c) an accepted validated intermediate endpoint (eg, large adenomatous polyps for colorectal prevention)
2. Evidence obtained from controlled trials without randomization with a, b, and c above
3. Evidence obtained from cohort or case-control analytic studies, preferably from more than one center or research group with a, b, and c above
4. Evidence obtained from multiple-time series with or without intervention with a, b, and c above
5. Ecologic (descriptive) studies (eg, international patterns studies, migration studies) with a, b, and c above
6. Opinions of respected authorities based on clinical experience or reports of expert committees (eg, any of the above study designs using nonvalidated surrogate endpoints)

Experimental trials are designed to correct for or eliminate selection, lead time, length, healthy volunteer, and other biases when prospectively testing a detection procedure to determine its effect on outcome. The highest level of evidence and greatest benefit is mortality reduction in a randomized controlled trial. For most sites, such evidence is not, and may never be, available. Theoretically it is possible, but the sample size that is needed, the expense, and the duration for such trials in many sites, such as melanoma or gastric cancers, make this approach impractical at present. Therefore, evidence obtained by other design methods is often used, or intermediate endpoints of intervention effect are employed.

Case-control and cohort studies provide indirect evidence for the effectiveness of primary prevention. Such studies do not prove a mortality reduction effect, but they can suggest a mortality reduction. However, the potential for bias to invalidate inferences from case-control and cohort studies must be recognized. Likewise, an intervention that decreases the incidence of invasive cancers or of colonic polyps may be suggestive evidence of efficacy.

Descriptive uncontrolled studies based on the experience of individual physicians, hospitals, and nonpopulation-based registries may yield some information on prevention.

Aerodigestive tract cancers (cancers of the head, neck, oral cavity, pharynx, larynx, esophagus, and lung) are a major problem, with 1994 mortality estimated at 172,000 deaths despite intensive efforts in primary prevention, screening, and therapy. Long-term survival rates have not improved substantially since the 1960s. Tobacco exposure is the dominant risk factor for aerodigestive cancers, especially for lung cancer. Tobacco use along with heavy alcohol consumption is a major risk factor for head, neck, and esophageal cancer.

There is strong evidence to show that avoidance of smoking and smoking cessation result in decreased mortality from primary aerodigestive cancers (evidence level 6). Evidence suggests that long-term smoking avoidance results in decreased incidence of second primary aerodigestive tumors (evidence level 3). Preliminary evidence suggests that chemopreventive approaches may reduce the incidence of second primary tumors in patients successfully treated for an initial head, neck, or lung cancer (evidence level 1). Preliminary evidence also suggests that chemoprevention using retinoids, and possibly natural agents such as carotenoids or vitamin E, suppresses or reverses premalignancy in individuals with oral leukoplakia, but not bronchial metaplasia (evidence levels 1 and 6).

Understanding the biology of carcinogenesis is crucial to the development of effective chemoprevention. Two basic concepts supporting chemoprevention are the multistep nature of carcinogenesis, which we have already mentioned (initiation, promotion, and progression, which for aerodigestive cancers might be leukoplakia, metaplasia, and dysplasia), associated with malignant transformation rates up to 30–40%; and the concept of field carcinogenesis. This concept proposes that multiple independent neoplastic lesions occurring within the aerodigestive field can result from repeated exposure to carcinogens such as tobacco. Patients who develop cancers of the aerodigestive tract secondary to cigarette smoke are also likely to have multiple premalignant lesions of independent origin within the carcinogen-exposed field. In addition, the use of chewing tobacco is a major risk factor for oral cancer. Avoidance of tobacco use and of heavy alcohol consumption are the most effective preventive measures. A recent study found that smoking cessation was significantly correlated with reversal of bronchial premalignancy (squamous metaplasia), suggesting that smoking cessation may halt the early stages of the carcinogenic process, but may have no effect on late stages of carcinogenesis.

Chemoprevention is defined as the use of specific natural or synthetic chemical agents to reverse, suppress, or prevent carcinogenesis before the development of invasive malignancy. It is not yet established in standard clinical practice and phase III studies are still ongoing. The field cancerization hypothesis has guided the development of these studies and early data show that 3 months of treatment with isotretinoin (13-cis-retinoic acid) can dramatically reverse oral leukoplakia. The activity of retinoids in the chemoprevention of lung cancer remains to be established in future trials. Adjuvant phase III trials of isotretinoin and etretinate (tegison) have demonstrated a marked reduction in the development of second primary tumors for patients treated with a retinoid following local therapy for head and neck cancer.

Colorectal cancer is the third most common malignant neoplasm worldwide and the second leading cause of cancer deaths (irrespective of gender) in the United States. The risk of colorectal cancer begins to increase after age 40 and rises sharply at the ages of 50–55; the risk doubles with each succeeding decade, reaching a peak by age 75. Despite advances in surgical technique and adjuvant therapy, there has been only a modest impact on patients who present with advanced neoplasms. Hence, effective primary and secondary preventive approaches are needed.

Epidemiologic, experimental (animal), and clinical investigations suggest that diets high in total fat, protein, calories, and alcohol, and low in calcium and dietary fiber, particularly that derived from vegetables, are associated with an increased incidence of colorectal cancer (evidence levels 3b and 5b). Nonsteroidal antiinflammatory drugs (NSAIDS), including sulindac and aspirin, may prevent adenoma formation or cause adenomatous polyps to regress (evidence level 1c). Cigarette smoking is associated with an increased tendency to form adenomas and develop colorectal cancer (evidence level 3b). Colonoscopy with removal of adenomatous polyps reduces the risk of colorectal cancer (evidence level 3a).

Primary prevention concerns the identification of genetic, biologic, and environmental factors that are etiologic or pathogenetic in the development of cancer and subsequent complete or significant interference with their effects on carcinogenesis. Removal of premalignant lesions (adenomas) may also be an effective form of primary prevention. The goal of secondary prevention, including screening of the general population and surveillance of high-risk populations, is the identification and appropriate management of preneoplastic and early neoplastic lesions. Dietary factors account for about 30% of the attributable risk. Although far from clear-cut, the available evidence suggests colorectal cancer risk is possibly associated with some interaction of dietary fat and protein and caloric intake. Most animal and epidemiologic studies show a protective effect of dietary fiber on colon carcinogenesis. The term *fiber* is used to describe a complex mixture of compounds including insoluble fiber (typified by wheat bran and cellulose) and soluble fiber (usually dried beans). Although there is some evidence of a protective effect of NSAIDS in colon cancer, not all studies showed it; in fact several large studies failed to show any such protective effect and there is some concern about the long-term risks of inducing GI ulceration. A sedentary lifestyle has been associated in some but not all studies with an increased risk of colorectal cancer. Five studies have reported a positive association between alcohol intake and colorectal adenomas. A positive association between current alcohol intake and adenomas was found to be limited to the larger adenomas, suggesting that alcohol intake could act at the promotional phase of the adenoma-carcinoma sequence. Most case-control studies of cigarette exposure and adenomas have found an elevated risk for smokers.

Skin cancer is the most commonly occurring cancer in the United States. It accounts for 1% of all cancer deaths in this country and appears to be increasing. Evidence suggests that reduction of exposure to ultraviolet (UV) radiation will reduce the incidence of nonmelanoma (basal cell and squamous cell) skin cancer. Sun exposure can be reduced by changing patterns of outdoor activities to reduce time of exposure to high-intensity UV radiation, and by using sunscreens or wearing protective clothing when exposed to sunlight (evidence levels 1c, 3b, and 6). For melanoma, the evidence suggests that avoidance of sunburns, especially in childhood and adolescence, may reduce the incidence of cutaneous melanoma. Sunburn can be avoided by changing patterns of outdoor activities to reduce time of exposure to high-intensity UV radiation, and by wearing protective clothing when exposed to sunlight. It is unknown whether sunscreens are protective for cutaneous melanoma (evidence levels 3b, 5b, and 6).

Most evidence about UV radiation exposure and the prevention of skin cancer comes from observational and analytic epidemiologic studies, not from experimental studies in humans. Such studies have consistently shown that increased cumulative sun exposure is a risk factor for nonmelanoma skin cancer. Individuals whose skin tans poorly or burns easily after sun exposure are particularly susceptible. One may conclude that if exposure to the sun is reduced, the result will be a reduced incidence of nonmelanoma skin cancer. However, it is not known if reduction of exposure to UV radiation through the use of sunscreens and/or protective clothing or through limitation of exposure time can reduce the incidence of nonmelanoma skin cancer in humans. The relationship between UV radiation exposure and cutaneous melanoma is less clear. Rather than cumulative sun exposure, it is intermittent acute sun exposure that seems to be more damaging; such exposures in childhood or adolescence may be particularly important. One animal study suggests that sunscreens that protect against sunburn may not protect against UV radiation–induced cutaneous melanoma.

16

GUIDELINES FOR THE CANCER-RELATED CHECKUP

When caring for a patient who has been treated for a specific malignancy, it is hoped that the guidelines in this book for the cancer involved will be helpful. In addition, the patient remains at least at the same risk, or more likely at increased risk, for developing a second malignant neoplasm, and will look to the physician for guidance in prevention and, failing that, early detection. The patient's family, now sensitized to the risks of cancer, may also consult the physician for similar guidance.

Prevention is discussed in chapter 15. Guidelines for the cancer-related checkup will be discussed here based on the recommendations of the American Cancer Society (ACS) (see Table 16-1). These guidelines, which have evolved and continue to change with new information, have recently been called into question by some contradictory recommendations of the National Cancer Institute (NCI) in regard to mammography for breast cancer and examinations for prostate cancer. The discrepancy is in part related to what the ACS and the NCI accept as valid evidence, and the perspective from which each group views the problem. Hopefully, such a discussion will help the clinician in the care and counseling of his or her patients.

To better understand the current recommendations, a brief review of their history and evolution will be helpful. During the 1970s, the ACS distributed a one-page chart which, among other recommendations, included an annual Pap smear for women over age 20, an annual chest x-ray for individuals at increased risk for lung cancer (primarily cigarette smokers and asbestos-exposed workers), an annual digital rectal examination, sigmoidoscopy, and stool guaiac test for persons over age 40, an annual mammogram for women over the age of 50, and one for women aged 40 to 49 if they or their mothers or sisters had breast cancer. These recommendations were based on a consensus of disease-specific task forces and a scientific and medical advisory board.

In 1978, the ACS decided to review its recommendations and to provide a more firm scientific basis for the guidelines. Its Service and Rehabilitation, Professional Education, and Medical and Scientific Committees were assisted by David M. Eddy, M.D., Ph.D., then medical policy analyst at Stanford University (later a professor at Duke University, and now writing from Jackson, Wyoming); the committees reviewed the world's literature, consulted experts, and finally submitted the findings to the ACS National Board of Directors, which published them (*Ca—A Cancer Journal for Clinicians*, 1980; 30:194–240).

The ACS made it clear that its major objectives were to detect cancer as early in its natural history as possible and to achieve the greatest possible reduction in morbidity and mortality. In doing so, its four major concerns were:

1. There must be good evidence that each test or procedure recommended is medically effective in reducing morbidity or mortality.
2. The medical benefits must outweigh the risks.
3. The cost of each test or procedure must be reasonable compared to its expected benefits.
4. Recommended actions must be practical and feasible.

It was emphasized that these recommendations pertain to the early detection of cancer—the search for early cancer in asymptomatic people on an individual basis. They were not recommendations for mass screening of large populations (not all of whom are necessarily asymptomatic) through a centrally coordinated program at public expense.

Two of the new 1980 recommendations elicited a stormy reaction. The chest x-ray was not recommended (nor was sputum cytology) and the Pap test was modified for women ages 20 to 65 from annually to "at least every 3 years after two negative examinations 1 year apart and more frequently in high-risk women (early age at first intercourse, multiple sex partners)." I vividly recall, as then president of the Connecticut division of ACS, that at the recommendation of our Professional Education Committee and at the direction of our Board of Directors, I wrote a critical letter to the National ACS office questioning the deletion of the routine annual chest x-ray and the

TABLE16-1. SUMMARY OF AMERICAN CANCER SOCIETY RECOMMENDATIONS FOR THE EARLY DETECTION OF CANCER IN ASYMPTOMATIC PEOPLE

Test or Procedure	Sex	Age	Frequency
Sigmoidoscopy, preferably flexible	M&F	50 and over	Every 3–5 years
Fecal occult blood test	M&F	50 and over	Every year
Digital rectal examination	M&F	40 and over	Every year
Prostate exam*	M	50 and over	Every year
Pap test	F	All women who are, or who have been, sexually active, or have reached age 18, should have an annual Pap test and pelvic examination. After a woman has had three or more consecutive satisfactory normal annual examinations, the Pap test may be performed less frequently at the discretion of her physician.	
Pelvic examination	F	18–40	Every 1–3 years with Pap test
		Over 40	Every year
Endometrial tissue sample	F	At menopause, if at high risk**	At menopause and thereafter the discretion of the physician
Breast self-examination	F	20 and over	Every month
Breast clinical examination	F	20–40	Every 3 years
		Over 40	Every year
Mammography***	F	40–49	Every 1–2 years
		50 and over	Every year
Health counseling and cancer checkup****	M&F	Over 20	Every 3 years
	M&F	Over 40	Every year

*Annual digital rectal examination and prostate-specific antigen should be performed on men 50 years and older. If either is abnormal, further evaluation should be considered.
**History of infertility, obesity, failure to ovulate, abnormal uterine bleeding, or unopposed estrogen or tamoxifen therapy.
***Screening mammography should begin by age 40.
****To include examination for cancers of the thyroid, testicles, ovaries, lymph nodes, oral region, and skin.
Revised November 1992.

modification of the Pap smear frequency. Similar letters from other states, from radiologic societies, and gynecologic societies were answered with a review of the then available scientific and medical literature upon which the recommendations were based. When passions cooled and there was time for reflection of the controversy on its scientific merits, it became clear to me and many (or most) others that the ACS had acted responsibly and in conformity with its objectives and concerns.

The NCI, through its online service, Physician's Data Query (PDQ), makes recommendations for screening based on its view that screening is a means of accomplishing early detection of disease in asymptomatic populations. Detection examinations, tests, or procedures used in screening are usually not diagnostic, but sort out persons suspicious for the presence of cancer from those who are not. Diagnosis is made following a work-up, a biopsy, or other tests in pursuing symptoms or positive detection procedures. Three requirements must be met for screening to be useful:

1. There must be a test or procedure that will detect cancers earlier.
2. There must be evidence that treatment at an earlier stage of disease will result in an improved outcome.
3. The prevalence of the detectable preclinical phase of the disease should be high enough among the persons being screened.

These requirements are necessary, but not sufficient, to prove the efficacy of screening. There are some cancers for which screening does not appear useful: those where no early detection tests exist, as in cancer of the pancreas; and in cancers with no apparent localized stage, as in leukemia. The relation of stage to survival and mortality is the basis of clinical cancer management. It is the major factor in prognosis, in the determination of treatment, and in the evaluation of end results. In the 1940s, a generalized staging classification of localized, regional, and distant (LRD) was developed to show long-term trends, and is still useful. The Surveillance, Epidemiology, and End Results (SEER) Program of the NCI gathers data from 11 geographic areas, covering approximately 10% of the United States population. These data, because of their population-based coverage in these areas and long duration (1973 to the present), are a unique and important resource in considering the potential for early cancer detection and for following tumor site–specific trends in incidence and mortality. Patients with localized cancers have a better survival than those with regional or distant spread. In considering more than a million cancers (excluding in situ carcinomas, and squamous and basal cell cancers of the skin) by stage, the 5-year relative survival rate is 78% for localized cancer, 45% for regional cancer, and 12% for distant metastatic cancer.

In the more detailed TNM system, which has been periodically modified, the (T)umor size, the status of the lymph (N)odes, and the status of distant (M)etastases are also categorized. These elements are then grouped into stages 0–IV according to their association with survival. As malignant tumors increase in size, they have a greater propensity to metastasize to regional lymph nodes and to distant sites. Stage has such a profound effect that all randomized treatment trials require the comparison of similar stages in evaluating differences in outcome.

Differences in outcome may be related to several biases that make interpretation of results difficult:

1. Lead-time bias is the average time by which the conventional diagnosis of cancer is advanced among the cases detected by screening. The lead-time factor makes it impossible to compare the survival experience of symptom-diagnosed cases directly with the survival of screen-detected cases, because what appears to be extended survival may be an artifact of earlier diagnosis. In fact, some claim that the earlier diagnosis only leads to more time to worry about the cancer if it is not curable.
2. Length bias is difficult to estimate. It results from the fact that slow-growing tumors, with a favorable prognosis, have a longer detectable preclinical phase than the rapidly growing lesion with an unfavorable prognosis.
3. Volunteer bias is the self-selection for screening by individuals who are concerned about their health and may have a higher incidence of tumors, or who are the type of people who take better care of themselves and will tend to do better no matter when they are diagnosed.
4. The "so what" bias applies to some small cancers that may never have surfaced in life and would not have caused any morbidity or mortality, yet may be detected by screening. Prostate cancer in the very elderly is a tumor that is frequently found at autopsy but caused no problems during life. An early diagnosis of such a cancer might give the patient grief with no benefit and might inflate the apparent survival without reducing mortality.

To evaluate the measures of an improved outcome, there are varying levels of evidence that support a given statement from the strongest evidence to just opinions:

1. Evidence obtained from at least one randomized controlled trial
2. Evidence obtained from controlled trials without randomization

3. Evidence obtained from cohort or case-controlled analytic studies, preferably from more than one center or research group
4. Evidence obtained from multiple time series with or without intervention
5. Opinions of respected authorities based on clinical experience, descriptive studies, or reports of expert committees

The recommendations are based on explicit evidence published in the literature.

With these criteria, we are in a better position to evaluate the ACS and NCI advice. In the current ACS recommendations, chest x-ray is simply not mentioned. The NCI screening summaries do not include lung cancer. Lung cancer prevention by the cessation of tobacco smoking has been a major objective of both organizations. The recommendation for the Pap smear has been modified to annual examinations, and after three consecutive satisfactory normal examinations, less frequently at the discretion of the woman's physician. The NCI recommendation is not in conflict and states: "Evidence strongly suggests a decrease in mortality from regular screening with Pap tests in women who are sexually active or have reached 18 years of age. The upper age limit at which to cease screening is unknown" (evidence levels 3, 4, and 5).

Although the 1980 guidelines did not recommend routine mammography for women ages 40–49, but only that these women "consult their physician," in 1983 the ACS modified the recommendation for women ages 40–49 to suggest a mammogram every 1–2 years. This was brought about by the publication of the first results of the Breast Cancer Detection Demonstration Project (BCDDP). The recommendation was reaffirmed after a joint consensus conference with the American College of Radiology in 1987, and again after a joint conference in October 1993 with the International Union Against Cancer (UICC). It was recognized that this frequency would be more expensive, but it was felt that it would increase early diagnosis, increase survival, and reduce morbidity.

In December 1993, the NCI executive committee voted to change its earlier recommendation on mammography, which had been the same as that of the ACS, to a recommendation to women ages 40–49 to discuss with a health professional the advisability of breast cancer screening with mammography, taking into account family history of breast cancer and other risk factors. The NCI also recommended annual clinical breast examination as a prudent practice for this group, in essence a suggestion that mammography not be done in that age group because there was no evidence that it decreased mortality. This position was reaffirmed in a Physician's Data Query (PDQ) summary dated October 31, 1994, stating: "There is insufficient evidence to make an informed decision regarding efficacy of screening in women ages 40–49 years. In the first 5–7 years of follow-up there is no reduction in mortality from breast cancer that can be attributed to screening; there is an uncertain and, if present, a marginal reduction in mortality at about 10–12 years; only one study provides information on long-term effects beyond 12 years, and more information is needed" (evidence levels 1, 2, 3, and 5).

This decision was made in spite of a November 1993 National Cancer Advisory Board (NCAB) vote of 14–1 recommending against the change and for retention of the previous NCI summary, which was essentially the same as the ACS guidelines on mammography. There is an extensive and growing literature on this controversy with editorials in peer-reviewed journals (including the *Journal of the NCI*), articles in newspapers, magazines, and particularly in women's magazines, and on radio and television talk shows. The public is confused and so are most doctors, so the advice to consult your physician may be of little value. The NCI defends its action on the basis of its claim that the decision was based solely on the preponderance of the evidence of eight randomized prospective trials that failed to show any reduction in mortality in the screened group. The proponents of the ACS recommendations counter that all the studies relied on were too small to show a statistically significant difference even if there were a 30% difference. In addition, the Canadian trial, the National Breast Screening Study (NBSS), upon which the greatest emphasis was placed by the NCI because it was the only one of the studies specifically designed to evaluate the 40–49 age group, was flawed. It has been suggested that the NBSS had poor mammography technique, radiologists not specifically trained in mammographic interpretation, and did not discount 17 women with known palpable breast masses and also failed to discount from the screened group those who were assigned to get mammograms but never actually did, or from the control group those who went outside the study and actually did have mammograms.

The controversy became political on October 20, 1994, when the Committee on Government Operations of the United States House of Representatives sent a report to Congress entitled "Misused Science: The National Cancer Institute's Elimination of Mammography Guidelines for Women in their Forties." The report criticized the NCI for ignoring the advice of the presidentially appointed NCAB, for a flawed review of the scientific data, and for the inability of the NCI to produce transcripts or records of the executive committee meeting at which the decision was made. The congressional report recommended that the NCI conduct a formal consensus conference on mammographic screening of younger women, consider data beyond randomized clinical trials like the BCDDP, conduct further research on the question, and until then adopt the statement from the October 1993 UICC meeting. The UICC statement, while acknowledging that the data are unclear, noted a slight advantage in survival among younger women who undergo mammography screening.

One may wonder how two such competent and respected groups can look at the same body of information and come to somewhat different conclusions. The NCI placed its emphasis only on evidence derived from randomized clinical trials that mainly happened to be performed in Canada, Sweden, and Scotland, and none in the United States, which has a more heterogeneous population with large minorities that the other countries do not have. The ACS relied on the United States studies by the Health Insurance Plan (HIP) of New York and on the BCDDP run by the ACS and NCI together in the United States, and considered benefits in addition to mortality reduction, such as opportunity for more conservative therapies as well as evidence for prolongation of survival.

The ACS recommendations were intended to be interim guidelines to be reviewed and updated as additional information became available. In November 1992, the ACS Board of Directors approved inclusion of early detection procedures for prostate cancer, a major change, involving a recommendation for the use of prostate-specific antigen (PSA) as part of the cancer-related checkup for men age 50 and over. This is not a recommendation for mass screening but an addition to the earlier recommendation for annual digital rectal examinations beginning at age 40. This recommendation was occasioned by the observation that prostatic cancer was becoming a more frequently diagnosed malignancy (largely due to the PSA), and indeed, by 1994 it surpassed both lung and breast cancer in incidence, so that it is now the most frequently diagnosed cancer in the United States. The recommendation was coupled with the observation that "while an examination for prostate carcinoma detects tumors at more favorable stages (anatomically less extensive disease), reduction in mortality from screening has not yet been documented." The NCI recommendation was that "there is insufficient evidence to establish that a decrease in mortality from prostate cancer occurs with screening by digital rectal examination, transrectal ultrasound, or serum markers including prostate-specific antigen" (evidence level 5). Other critics suggested that early diagnosis was irrelevant because asymptomatic patients with prostate carcinoma should not be treated because they have a long survival anyway and some will die with, but not because of, their prostate cancer. The available evidence, however, suggests that most cases of early detection with PSA are not the cancers that would remain asymptomatic until death, but rather slowly progressive cancers that would become symptomatic in time and eventually lead to mortality if not treated, unless the patient dies of some other cause before the prostatic cancer becomes morbid. The question of cost effectiveness remains controversial, but ACS and the American Urologic Association (AUA) still feel that PSA is a useful test in the cancer checkup.

Additional revised ACS recommendations were for evaluation of endometrial carcinoma with a tissue sample at menopause for women at high risk, ie, those with a history of infertility, obesity, failure to ovulate, abnormal uterine bleeding, or unopposed estrogen or tamoxifen therapy. This subject is not very controversial.

The new recommendations for the early detection of colorectal cancer in asymptomatic people involve a sigmoidoscopy (preferably flexible), for males and females age 50 and over, every 3–5 years (or they note, at even longer intervals), based on the advice of a physician. The term *fecal occult blood* was substituted for *stool guaiac slide test*, so that the current recommendation is for a fecal occult blood test every year for males and females age 50 and over. The NCI recommendations are similar.

Additional cancer sites considered by the NCI with no recommendations from the ACS include gastric, ovarian, testicular, skin, and oral cancer. The NCI recommendations are:

1. For gastric cancer there is insufficient evidence to establish that screening would result in a decrease in mortality in the U.S. population.
2. For ovarian cancer there is insufficient evidence to establish that screening with serum markers, such as CA-125 levels, transvaginal ultrasound, or pelvic examinations would result in a decrease in mortality (evidence levels 4 and 5).
3. For testicular cancer there is insufficient evidence to establish that screening results in a decrease in mortality (evidence level 5).
4. For skin cancer there is evidence from epidemiologic studies to establish that a decrease in mortality occurs with routine examination of the skin (evidence level 5).
5. For oral cancer there is insufficient evidence to establish that screening results in a decrease in mortality (evidence level 5).

When the recommendations of the ACS and NCI are similar—colorectal, lung (no recommendation), and cervical cancers—the decision of what to do is easy. Where only one or the other has a recommendation—gastric, ovarian, testicular, skin, oral, and endometrial cancers—the decision is easy. When the recommendations are different, as for breast mammography for the 40–49 age group and for prostate cancer, the physician will have to decide for himself or herself.

If I were a health care bureaucrat concerned with mass screening and cost containment, I would follow the NCI guidelines, which were developed with the idea of mass screening in mind. As a taxpayer, I would applaud such a decision. If I were a clinician whose primary concern was the welfare of the individual patient under my care, I would prefer to resolve doubtful data and derivative practices to err on the side of the safety of my patient. Thus, as a clinician, I would follow the current ACS guidelines, recognizing that they are interim guidelines subject to revision as new information becomes available. Although the ACS recommendations are more costly than the NCI recommendations, the ACS believes that they will prolong quality of life survival, and in most cases, reduce mortality.

17

TUMOR MARKERS

In the broadest sense of the term, a tumor marker could be anything associated with a malignancy that indicates its presence, quantity, future behavior, or even the risk of its development. Thus, the history of exposure to specific chemicals or the smoking of tobacco may be tumor markers, especially for lung, bladder, or larynx cancer. A physical finding such as a lump in the axilla or a fungating mass in the breast may be a tumor marker, as could cytology of exfoliated cells from sputum, urine, or cervical brushings. Biomarkers, like chromosomal translocations, oncogenes, other gene markers, etc, are being studied for their predictive value as tumor markers. For this discussion, we will limit ourselves to a consideration of circulating tumor-associated markers present in serum, plasma, or urine.

Tumor markers may be of use in:

1. Screening for malignancy in asymptomatic or high-risk populations
2. Finding individuals suspected of having an undiagnosed malignancy
3. Prognosis of the probable course of a malignancy
4. Predicting recurrence of a neoplasm after primary therapy

We will further restrict the scope of the subject to solid tumors, primarily in adults, for which commercially available tests have been evaluated to some extent.

To be ideally useful, tumor markers should be:

1. Sensitive—they should be abnormal in all or a very high proportion of patients with the neoplasm in question.
2. Specific—they should be negative in all or the vast majority of patients without the specific neoplasm.
3. Quantitative—the degree of abnormality of the marker should correlate with the mass or growth rate of the neoplasm.
4. Economic—they should be relatively low in cost, ie, cost-effective.
5. Safe—they should not cause morbidity, pain, or gross inconvenience.
6. Timely—they should detect the malignancy in its early phase before it becomes metastatic or clinically evident.
7. Relevant—they should be useful in significant clinical disorders that are common enough to matter and in which the untreated neoplasm results in morbidity or mortality.
8. Therapeutically important—they should detect the tumor at a stage in which early treatment can contribute to the patient's well-being by reducing morbidity and mortality.

These criteria are particularly important for early detection or screening. Since sensitivity and specificity are inversely related and far from 100% accurate in all tumor markers, increasing sensitivity will detect more true positives but will reduce specificity and will result in more false positives in patients who do not have cancer. These individuals will then need a costly and uncomfortable diagnostic evaluation to rule out the suspected neoplasm, and will endure the anxiety associated with a cancer diagnosis until it is ruled out. In some, the anxiety may persist because of their doubts that the new tests have definitively ruled it out.

Unfortunately, there is no clear-cut evidence that any tumor marker comes close enough to our ideal criteria to qualify at this time for routine clinical screening. Some that have been used in follow-up (f/u) or diagnosis of cancer are listed in Table 17-1 with the tumors or disorders in which they are abnormal. The closest tumor marker to even approach the criteria is the prostate-specific antigen (PSA) and its role is very controversial.

PSA is a glycoprotein isolated from human prostate extracts and seminal fluid. It is elevated in benign prostatic hypertrophy (BPH), prostatitis, and prostate cancer (CaPr). Even when the test is adequately sensitive and specific, and detects an early case of true CaPr, it may not be useful

TABLE 17-1. COMMON TUMOR MARKERS

Type	Tumor marker	Useful in cancer f/u	Elevated but not useful
Oncofetal antigens	CEA	colon, stomach, biliary (?) breast	lung, pancreas cirrhosis, COPD, smokers
	AFP	liver, testes	hepatitis, cirrhosis, pregnancy, IBD
Hormones	serotonin catecholamines	carcinoid pheochromocytoma neuroblastoma	
	calcitonin	medullary thyroid cancer	small-cell lung cancer
	HCG	choriocarcinoma, testicular	colon, melanoma, small-cell cancer
Tumor antigens	CA-125	ovary, endometrium	colon, lung, cirrhosis
	CA–15-3	(?) breast	ovary, lung
	CA–19-9	(?) pancreas	colon
	PSA	prostate	BPH, prostatitis
Enzymes	PAP	(?) prostate	
	LDH	lymphoma	benign liver, muscle, heart
Immunoglobulins	"M-spike"	myeloma, macroglobulinemia	

Abbreviations: CEA = carcinoembryonic antigen; AFP = alpha-fetoprotein; HCG = human chorionic gonadotropin; PSA = prostate-specific antigen; PAP = prostatic acid phosphatase; LDH = lactic dehydrogenase; BPH = benign prostatic hypertrophy; IBD = inflammatory bowel disease; COPD = chronic obstructive pulmonary disease.

according to some authors. They suggest that early CaPr is best treated by observation, sometimes for several years, before it shows itself to be aggressive enough to warrant specific therapy—chemical, hormonal, surgical, or radiation.

On the other side of the controversy, the American Cancer Society (ACS), the American Urologic Association (AUA), and most urologists believe that routine annual screening for early prostate cancer in men 50 years or older (perhaps up to age 70 or 75), along with an annual digital rectal examination, is worthwhile and will promote discovery of otherwise unsuspected early but serious cancer in asymptomatic men on an individual basis before metastasis occurs or the tumor becomes too bulky to safely and easily remove with acceptable morbidity. They contend that the tumors detected by this approach are not the small latent cancers that are found at autopsy and never cause clinical problems, but rather tumors that are destined to grow and metastasize and kill if not appropriately treated.

If the PSA is an isolated abnormality and only slightly elevated, it is probably best followed with a repeat examination after several months to see if it is rising and measure its rate of increase. A rapidly rising PSA, especially in association with a prostatic nodule, is an indication for a transrectal ultrasound (TRUS) and/or needle biopsy. While this procedure may detect CaPr at an earlier and more favorable stage (anatomically less extensive disease), and result in prolongation of survival, a clear reduction in mortality has not yet been documented and the procedure is not felt to be cost-effective. Hence, the National Cancer Institute (NCI) and many authors do not advocate PSA screening.

It is generally agreed that the PSA is a valuable adjunct in the diagnosis and f/u of CaPr. Indeed, after primary therapy has reduced the PSA to near normal levels, a significantly rising level is almost a sure sign of recurrence and should alert the physician to document the recurrence and consider possible additional therapy. None of the other tumor markers in Table 17-1 have even been suggested as useful in screening, but they may be helpful in both diagnosis and f/u of some neoplasms.

Carcinoembryonic antigen (CEA) is a glycoprotein found in embryonic tissue and postnatally in glandular cells of colon, rectum, stomach, bile ducts, and pancreas. It is elevated in cancers of the colon, rectum, stomach, bile ducts, pancreas, breast, lung, and in liver metastases from these sites. However, it is also elevated in cirrhosis of the liver, chronic obstructive pulmonary disease (COPD), and in some smokers. CEA is useful in f/u of carcinoma of the colon, rectum, stomach, and extrahepatic bile ducts. It is not generally considered useful in f/u of lung cancer because its ratio of sensitivity/specificity in that cancer is not good. In the f/u of pancreatic cancer, CEA's elevation is not early enough for any useful therapeutic interventions at this time. Although CEA is not generally thought to be cost-effective in f/u of breast cancer, many medical oncologists use it in f/u of high-risk patients based on their own experience.

Alpha-fetoprotein (AFP) is a glycoprotein that is produced in fetal liver and may be detected normally in very low concentrations after birth. It is significantly elevated in 80% of cases of hepatocellular carcinoma and in about 70% of patients with nonseminomatous testicular carcinoma, and is very important in the diagnosis and f/u of both of these tumors. The AFP level falls with successful therapy and rises with recurrence. It is sometimes elevated in hepatitis, cirrhosis, pregnancy, and inflammatory bowel disease, but this is rarely a problem in the f/u situation since the levels in malignancy are much higher or the benign condition is easily distinguished.

Human chorionic gonadotropin (HCG) is a glycoprotein normally produced by syncytiotrophoblast cells of the placenta during pregnancy and forms the basis of most urinary and serum pregnancy tests. It is elevated in almost all tumors of placental origin (choriocarcinoma, hydatidiform moles) and in 60% of men with nonseminomatous testicular carcinomas (NSTC). It is now generally detected by its beta-chain antigen, ie, beta-HCG. Its level correlates well with tumor burden in gestational trophoblastic disease and in NSTC, and can be used to guide therapy. A falling level after therapy indicates response, a stable level indicates residual disease, and a rising level indicates recurrence or progression.

CA-125 is a glycoprotein antigen defined by a monoclonal antibody against human ovarian carcinoma cells that is present in some fetal tissues but not in normal ovaries. It is elevated in 80% of women with ovarian cancer, but may also be elevated in pregnancy, pelvic inflammatory disease (PID), cirrhosis, endometriosis, uterine fibroids, pancreatitis, renal failure, some benign conditions that involve the peritoneal membranes, and in cancers of the lung, breast, colon, and endometrium. It is most useful in f/u of ovarian carcinoma and is occasionally useful in f/u of endometrial cancer. Persistent elevation after surgery is almost invariably associated with residual disease, but a normal level may be found in about half the patients who have some residual disease. A rising level is usually an indicator of recurrence.

CA-15-3 is a glycoprotein antigen defined by a monoclonal antibody produced against human milk fat globule membranes. It is elevated in patients with carcinoma of the breast, ovary, or lung, but has been used primarily in the f/u of breast cancer. Approximately 40–50% of patients who will develop metastases will have a preceding rise in either CEA or CA–15-3. However, the clinical utility of predicting impending relapse is not clear. Hence, most authors consider CA–15-3 investigational at this time, although many medical oncologists use it in f/u of high-risk patients.

CA–19-9 is a glycoprotein antigen defined by a monoclonal antibody originally derived from mice immunized with human colon carcinoma cells. The CA–19-9 epitope is normally present in cells of the biliary tract and is elevated with acute and chronic diseases of the biliary tract. It is also elevated in pancreatic cancer, biliary tract cancer, and less frequently in gastric and colorectal cancers. It has been used in f/u of pancreatic cancer and rises with recurrence. It is not cost-effective to follow it because by the time the recurrence is diagnosed, there is little useful further therapy.

Prostatic acid phosphatase is an enzyme secreted by normal prostate tissue. Abnormal levels indicate that a tumor has extended beyond the prostatic capsule. The enzyme elevation is late and does not correlate well with the body burden of CaPr, so it has been largely replaced by the PSA in diagnosis and f/u of CaPr.

Other tumor markers include the serotonin metabolite, 5-hydroxyindole acetic acid (5-HIAA), which is useful in the diagnosis and f/u of carcinoid; catecholamines, which are useful in the diagnosis and f/u of pheochromocytoma and neuroblastoma; and calcitonin, which is useful in f/u of medullary carcinoma of the thyroid. The other markers in Table 17-1 are well known and need no special commentary.

18

METASTASIS

Although some cancers kill by local growth in a vital location (eg, brain tumors or biliary duct tumors) and others do so by local interference with no extension (eg, head and neck tumors obstruct the airway or prevent oral food intake), most cause death by distant spread—metastasis. Accordingly, it is important to understand the process of metastasis, the pathways of metastasis, the likely location of most metastases, and the anticipated responses to metastases.

While we tend to think of metastasis simply as a malignant cell breaking off a primary neoplasm and establishing itself in the first capillary bed it encounters, as suggested by James Ewing in 1928, in fact, it is a much more complex process. It is estimated that fewer than one in 100,000 cells that uncouple from the primary neoplasm survive to form a metastasis. The metastatic phenomenon has been studied intensively, and is described as an eight-step process[1]:

1. Transformation of a normal cell to the neoplastic phenotype and its growth into a clone of malignant cells
2. Vascularization to allow further tumor mass growth
3. Cell mobilization and invasion into the host stroma, lymphatics, capillaries, and venules
4. Embolization (transport) in the circulation
5. Survival in the circulation despite interaction with host immune mechanisms, lymphocytes, macrophages, NK (natural killer) cells, mechanical stress, toxicity of high oxygen levels in the circulation, etc
6. Arrest in a distant capillary bed with adherence in a platelet-fibrin mesh
7. Extravasation into the organ's parenchyma with the establishment of a favorable microenvironment
8. Growth into a metastasis of often heterogeneous cells

That the host plays a crucial role in the metastatic process was first pointed out by Sir James Paget in 1889 with his "soil and seed" hypothesis. He suggested that metastasis is not a random process, and that the malignant cell, "the seed," might go to many sites, but would grow only in an environmentally suitable site, "the soil." It has been estimated that during tumor surgery (depending on site, size, and manipulation of the tumor) about 100 million tumor cells are released into the circulation, but very few metastases are detected in both human and animal studies. In animal studies where viable malignant cells are injected into the circulation, on the average only 1% form tumor nodules. Thus, both theories are correct: malignant cells will grow only in suitable sites; but they will not grow there if they do not get there. A few of the more common pathways of metastasis[2,3] are depicted in Figures 18-1 and 18-2.

Primary tumors with a high incidence of metastases are as follows:

colon and rectum	kidney
prostate	melanoma (depth > 2.26 mm)
lung	primary bone
stomach	childhood solid tumors
breast (stage II or III)	testis, nonseminoma
pancreas	bladder, high-grade, invasive

Intra-abdominal primary tumors tend to metastasize via the mesenteric lymphatics and the portal venous system into the liver, which is a favorable environment for supporting metastases. From the liver, these tumors can metastasize to the lung (see Figure 18-1). Liver metastases occur principally as a site of drainage if the gastrointestinal (GI) tract or its serosa are primarily or secondarily involved.

170

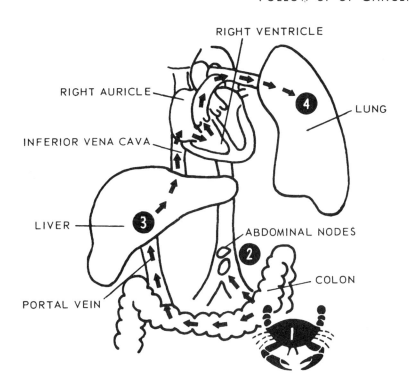

FIGURE 18-1. A carcinoma of the large bowel (1) usually metastasizes to mesenteric and para-aortic lymph nodes (2); it may also reach the liver through the portal veins (3), the right heart through the inferior vena cava, and through the pulmonary arteries, the lung (4). (Reproduced with permission from *Patterns of Metastases,* by H. A. Gilbert, 1979. © 1979 Adria Laboratories, Inc.)

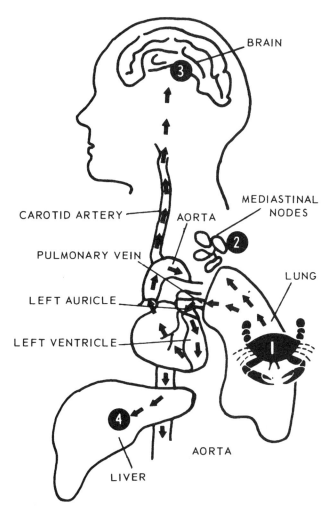

FIGURE 18-2. A bronchial carcinoma (1) usually metastasizes to mediastinal lymph nodes (2). Through pulmonary veins, it may reach the left auricles and ventricles. Once in the arterial circulation, it often goes to the brain (3) and also the liver (4). (Reproduced with permission from *Patterns of Metastases,* by H. A. Gilbert, 1979. © 1979 Adria Laboratories, Inc.)

Breast cancer with one or more positive axillary nodes will be metastatic in 53% of cases, and with four or more positive nodes in 80% of cases within 5 years. For patients without involvement of axillary nodes at surgery there will be 21% recurrence overall, and less for those with small primary tumors. Breast cancer metastasizes to the lung via the lymph nodes and superior vena cava and to the bony skeleton via the intercostal veins, with or without nodal involvement. Liver involvement, although common at autopsy, occurs much later in the course of the disease. Metastases may arrive there via the pleural lymphatics transdiaphragmatically or simply via the arterial circulation from the lung. It was once thought that adenocarcinoma spread via the lymphatics and sarcoma via the blood vascular system. They are widely interconnected and it is now realized that metastases can follow both pathways, although particular tumors have characteristic patterns of spread. Early breast cancer usually travels via the regional lymph nodes and later spreads to organs, but 25% of early spread is hematogenous with no known lymph node involvement.

The term "early" is really a misnomer. A tumor nodule with 0.5-cm diameter that is barely detectable radiologically is composed of about 100 million malignant cells and has already undergone 27 doublings. By the time it is palpable at 1 cm, it will have undergone 30 doublings and been present for 2 to 10 years. By 35 to 40 doublings, the tumor will be 100 to 1000 grams and, and in most cases, lethal. Tumors are not only heterogeneous in their doubling time, but frequently in their histology as well. Hence, when they respond to therapy, one population may respond well, whereas another population in the same tumor may be relatively resistant and may itself metastasize. Cells able to successfully metastasize may represent a small subpopulation of cells (0.01%) within a tumor and they may emerge long before the tumor is detectable radiographically or by palpation. A tumor has a greater probability of metastasis if it is poorly difffferentiated, has many mitoses present (a sign of a rapid doubling time), and is of specific histologic type with a tendency to early metastasis (eg, small-cell carcinoma of the lung). When they do metastasize, tumor cells seem to grow better in orthotopic sites and are more likely to seed to them than to ectopic sites. In addition, secondaries often have shorter doubling times than primaries and therefore grow faster and are prone to tertiary and quaternary metastases to additional sites.

Primary tumors with a low incidence of metastasis are:

brain	cervix
head and neck	melanoma (depth < 0.76 mm)
breast (stage I)	thyroid (especially papillary)
bladder, low-grade, superficial	seminoma

As a general principle, very few tumor cells that are released ultimately form metastatic foci in the immunocompetent host. The bloodstream seems to be a hostile environment for cancer cells shed from a solid tumor. Lymphatics with their slower circulations provide a more suitable environment. Even so, most of the tumor cells are killed in the lymphatic circulation. Some remain viable and grow in the draining lymph nodes or are passed through into the venous circulation, either by lymphaticovenous communications or through the thoracic ducts. Some tumor metastases, like breast and melanoma, can remain viable but dormant in the body for 30 years and then grow. Lymph nodes may serve as a repository for later dissemination. Thoracic duct drainage is into the jugular trunk, then to the superior vena cava, the right heart, the pulmonary arteries, and the lung. Once a metastasis is established in the lung, it has access to the arterial circulation just as does a primary lung tumor. This is one of the explanations for metastases to the brain, heart muscle, eye, thyroid, skin, etc (see Figure 18-2).

Another pathway for spread, especially to form bone metastases, is the vertebral vein system that communicates with the caval venous systems, the paravertebral systems to the bones and skull, and through these sinusoidal systems to the arterial circulation without direct access to the heart, Batson's paravertebral venous plexus (see Figure 18-3). This is a prime metastatic pathway for breast and prostate metastases to bone.

Serous cavities frequently form a pathway for spread as the proteinaceous fluids float tumor cell to distant parts. Ovarian tumors are often found, as ascitic tumors spread extensively throughout the peritoneal cavity, especially on the undersurface of the diaphragm and on the liver

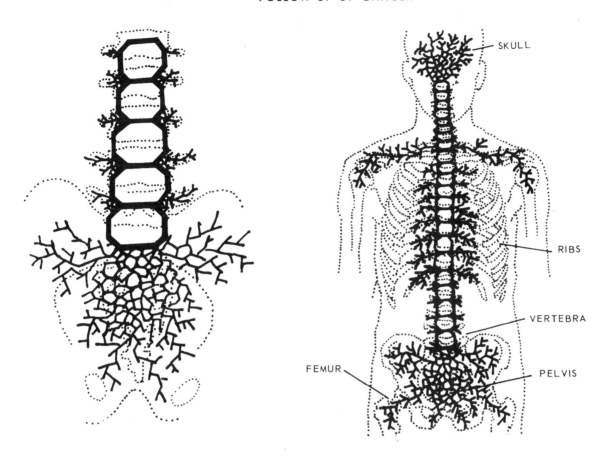

FIGURE 18-3. Batson's paravertebral venous plexus is a two-way thoroughfare frequently used by carcinoma of the prostate, breast, adrenals, and others, and is responsible for most of the bone metastases in these malignancies. (Reproduced with permission from *Patterns of Metastases*, by H. A. Gilbert, 1979. © 1979 Adria Laboratories, Inc.)

surface. Pancreatic tumors, appendiceal pseudomyxomas, gastric carcinomas, lymphomas, and endometrial carcinomas can also form as ascites and spread by this route. The thoracic cavity can spread lung, pleural, and breast tumors through the pleural fluid. Some tumors can spread by way of cerebrospinal fluid, including ependymomas, medulloblastomas, lymphomas, melanomas, and neuroblastomas.

Most metastases are ultimately to the lung, liver, or bone (see Figure 18-4). Based on autopsy studies as well as clinical studies, the sources of liver, lung, bone, and brain metastases are:

BONE	BRAIN
prostate	lung
breast	melanoma
Ewing's sarcoma	secondary tumors from lung
thyroid	
bladder	
lung	
unknown primary	
neuroblastoma	

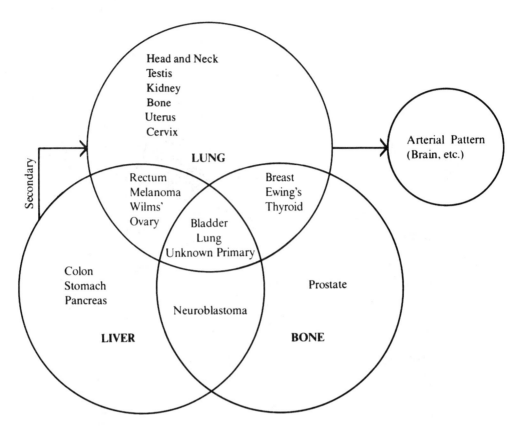

FIGURE 18-4. Primary clinically important metastatic patterns. (Reproduced with permission from *Patterns of Metastases*, by H. A. Gilbert, 1979. © 1979 Adria Laboratories, Inc.)

LIVER	LUNG
colon	breast
stomach	lung
pancreas	ovary
rectum	uterus
melanoma	bladder
gallbladder	kidney
bladder	testis
ovary	bone
uterus	melanoma
Wilms' tumor	Wilms' tumor
unknown primary	sarcomas
lung	unknown primary
breast	cervix
kidney	gastrointestinal
	secondary tumors from liver

There is a group of unusual metastases whose pattern is not clearly defined. Skin metastases have been noted from the lung, colon, bladder, kidney, cervix, ovary, and esophagus. Metastases to the GI tract tend to come from the lung, breast, ovary, cervix, and melanoma. Eye metastases arise from the breast, lung, melanoma, and esophagus. Myocardial metastases come from melanoma, lung, kidney, and leiomyosarcoma. Kidney metastases have been documented from the lung, breast, melanoma, and esophagus. Thyroid metastases may come from lymphomas and the lung.

In spite of the difficulties posed by late diagnosis, heterogeneity, and tumor mass, metastasis is potentially vulnerable. Failure to proceed through the eight-step process previously described can break the link in the metastatic chain and abort a metastasis. Tumors smaller than 1 to 2 mm receive all nutrients by simple diffusion, but progressive growth requires establishment of an adequate blood supply. Tumor vascularization is mediated by many angiogenic factors that are produced by the malignant cells and the host.[4] Without these angiogenic factors, blood vessels will not grow into the tumor, and with insufficient nutrition, the tumor cells necrose and die. At least eight angiogenic polypeptides have been identified and cloned. Many mechanisms are still undefined, but enough is known to begin to develop new anti-angiogenic therapies. Most of the inhibitors work by preventing vascular endothelial cells from responding to angiogenic factors, or inhibiting the production or release of angiogenic molecules or neutralizing these molecules in the bloodstream.

At least 11 angiogenesis inhibitors have now been described and the number is growing. A monoclonal antibody against basic fibroblastic growth factor, an important angiogenic polypeptide, has been developed and is being tested to inhibit angiogenesis and tumor growth. Angiogenesis inhibitors have potential as independent cancer drugs and are also being evaluated in combination with conventional chemotherapy used in tandem.

In addition to anti-angiogenic therapy, study of the increasing density of microvessels in tumors has indicated that active neovascularization is an independent and highly significant prognostic indicator for overall and relapse-free survival for prostate cancer, lung cancer, and node-positive and node-negative breast cancer. This provides some hope that further understanding of angiogenesis will lead to a better way to predict metastatic potential, and to treat a broad range of metastatic malignant neoplasms with anti-angiogenic substances to prolong survival and produce cures of a broad range of cancers.

References

1. Fidler IJ, Critical factors in the biology of human cancer metastases: Twenty-eighth GHA Clowes Memorial Award Lecture. Cancer Res 1990;50:6130.
2. del Regato JA, Pathways of metastatic spread of malignant tumors. Semin Oncol 1977;4:33.
3. Gilbert HA, Patterns of metastases. Columbus, OH: Adria Laboratories, 1979.
4. Folkman J, How is blood vessel growth regulated in normal and neoplastic tissue? Twenty-fourth GHA Clowes Memorial Award Lecture. Cancer Res 1986;46:467.

19

THE LATE TOXICITY OF CANCER THERAPY

In the treatment of cancer, three major modalities are used: surgery, radiation, and chemotherapy. Each has its benefits and liabilities, and we utilize them, consciously or subconsciously, based on estimates of cost-benefit ratios. The immediate toxicities are well known, but we often forget or do not know the late toxicity of some of the modalities we use.

The consequences of surgery are fairly obvious: loss of a limb or organ, impairment of function(s), scarring at the operative site, and the need for a prosthesis in some cases (artificial arm, leg, etc, breast implant, or need for reconstruction, etc, colostomy, ureterostomy, gastrostomy, etc). We sometimes forget the less obvious late effects like decreased immune competence after splenectomy, or the delayed (and controversial) effects of silicone breast prostheses, or the greater tendency for infection at sites of foreign body implantation.

The immediate effects of radiation therapy (RT) are erythema, pruritis, swelling, and local tissue destruction at the therapy site. Systemic toxicity includes nausea, vomiting, diarrhea, mucositis, stomatitis; marrow suppression with leukopenia, anemia, and thrombocytopenia; hair loss; profound fatigue and anorexia. These generally improve with time in most cases.

The late consequences of RT include late secondary malignancies; acute or chronic myelogenous leukemia 3 to 7 years or even 12 years later; solid malignancies 15 to 30 years and even 40 years later, especially involving the breast, lung, stomach, thyroid, and connective tissues. The risk of RT-induced solid neoplasms is particularly high under the age of 10 years. Overall, it has been estimated that 5% of second neoplasms are due to ionizing radiation. This is one reason for considering another therapeutic modality if it can give equivalent results at lesser toxicity and even for using MRI instead of CT imaging when either will give equally useful information. However, they frequently do not give equivalent information and the clinician will have to weigh the cost-benefit ratios in consultation with the radiologist when choosing between them and when deciding on their frequency of usage.

Nonmalignant late toxicities of RT include cataracts and dry eye syndrome; permanent xerostomia, dental caries, taste change or loss; bone necrosis, scoliosis, and growth retardation (especially in children); skin fibrosis, necrosis, telangiectasia, and permanent alopecia; pulmonary fibrosis and insufficiency (especially when used in conjunction with chemotherapy [CT] with bleomycin, methotrexate, carmustine, and busulfan); GI strictures and malabsorption; radiation nephritis; vaginal stenosis, dyspareunia, ovarian insufficiency with infertility and sterility; testicular insufficiency with sterility and often with impotence; hypothyroidism, pituitary insufficiency, and hypothalamic changes; loss of muscle bulk with fibrosis; chronic pericarditis and fibrosis, cardiomyopathy (especially when RT is used in conjunction with anthracycline CT); liver insufficiency and fibrosis (especially when RT is used in conjunction with CT with an anthracycline); long-term marrow impairment after total-body RT; radiation myelitis, impaired cognition, and learning disabilities (especially when RT is used with systemic methotrexate); lymphedema with swelling of arms and legs (especially when RT is used after lymphadenectomy). Other late sequelae are less common, and there may be some we have not yet recognized.

Delayed and Late Toxicity of Chemotherapy

It is well recognized that CT has many side effects of greater or lesser consequence. Acute toxicities are well known and the most important are bone marrow depression, nausea, vomiting, diarrhea, mucositis, stomatitis, rash, fever, hair loss, anaphylaxis, tissue necrosis due to vesicant drug extravasation, drowsiness, dizziness, and confusion. These are generally seen on the day of therapy or in the following week(s) and are handled by the treating medical oncologist.

Less well known are the delayed toxicities that are seen a month or more after therapy or the late toxicities that occur months or even years later. It is important for the primary physician to recognize them in order to ameliorate their symptoms and improve the patient's quality of life. The toxicities of standard drugs are listed in readily available textbooks, handbooks, and manuals of oncology and CT (see Bibliography). To help identify the probably offending drugs, since many patients do not know or recall the specific drugs they received, the listing of toxicities in Table 19-1 is by organ or system primarily affected. Recognition of the agent that caused one toxicity may alert the physician to other toxicities of the same drug, which if discerned early, may be ameliorated. Drugs are listed by their official generic name. The list is neither complete nor does it reflect degrees of severity or incidence. There may be some difference of opinion whether a toxicity is acute, late, or truly delayed.

TABLE 19-1. CHEMOTHERAPY SUSPECTED OF CAUSING TOXICITY TO ORGANS OR SYSTEMS

Organ or system	Toxicity	Suspected drugs
Auditory	Hearing loss, tinnitus	Cisplatin, carboplatin
Bladder	Hemorrhagic cystitis	Cyclophosphamide, ifosfamide, mitotane
Bone marrow	Prolonged pancytopenia	Alkylating agents (altretamine, busulfan, carmustine, chlorambucil, carboplatin, cisplatin, cyclophosphamide, dacarbazine, ifosfamide, lomustine, mechlorethamine, melphalan, mitomycin, procarbazine, streptozocin, thiotepa); intercalating agents (dactinomycin, daunorubicin, doxorubicin, idarubicin, mitoxantrone)
Bone, joint, muscle	Arthralgia, myalgia	Cytarabine, levamisole, paclitaxel, pentostatin
Cardiovascular	Cardiomyopathy	Daunorubicin, doxorubicin, idarubicin, mitoxantrone
	Raynaud's phenomenon	Bleomycin, cisplatin
Eye	Cataracts	Busulfan, mitotane
	Corneal changes and retinopathy	Tamoxifen
	Optic atrophy	Vincristine
	Visual disturbances	Altretamine, fludarabine, mitotane, tamoxifen
Hematopoietic	Agranulocytosis	Levamisole
	Coagulation defects	Asparaginase, plicamycin
	Hemolytic-uremic syndrome	Mitomycin
Kidney	Nephrogenic diabetes insipidus	Streptozocin
	Nephrotic syndrome	Aldesleukin
	Renal toxicity	Carboplatin, cisplatin, dacarbazine, fludarabine, interferon, lomustine, methotrexate, mitomycin, mitoxantrone, pentostatin, plicamycin, streptozocin
Liver	Cirrhosis, fibrosis, necrosis	Chlorambucil, cytarabine, dacarazine, etretinate, floxuridine, flutamide, mercaptopurine, methotrexate, mitomycin, mitoxantrone, plicamycin, streptozocin, thioguanine
	Veno-occlusive disease	Busulfan, carmustine

(Table continued on overleaf)

TABLE 19-1 (CONT'D.)

Organ or system	Toxicity	Suspected drugs
Lung	Pulmonary fibrosis, infiltrates, insufficiency	Bleomycin, busulfan, carmustine, chlorambucil, cyclophosphamide, estramustine, fludarabine, lomustine, melphalan, methotrexate, mitomycin, pentostatin, procarbazine
Nervous system	Ataxia	Altretamine
	Cerebellar ataxia	Fluorouracil
	Encephalopathy	Aldesleukin, cytarabine, fludarabine, methotrexate (with RT)
	Neuropsychiatric disorders	Aldesleukin, asparaginase, flutamide, ifosfamide, pentostatin, plicamycin, tamoxifen
	Peripheral neuropathy	Altretamine, carboplatin, cisplatin, cytarabine, paclitaxel, procarbazine, teniposide, vinblastine, vincristine
	Pseudotumor cerebri	Etretinate
Ovary	Diminished function, amenorrhea, infertility	Alkylating agents, methotrexate
	Masculinization	Aminoglutethimide
Pancreas	Pancreatitis	Asparaginase, cytarabine
Second malignancies	Acute myelogenous leukemia	Alkylating agents, etoposide, teniposide
	Solid tumors—bladder cancer	Cyclophosphamide, ifosfamide
Skin and appendages	Extravasation injury	Carmustine, dactinomycin, daunorubicin, doxorubicin, idarubicin, mechlorethamine, mitomycin, mitoxantrone, plicamycin, vinblastine, vincristine
	Hyperkeratosis	Bleomycin
	Hyperpigmentation	Bleomycin, busulfan, daunorubicin, doxorubicin, fluorouracil
Systemic	Drug fever	Aminoglutethimide
Fetus	Teratogenesis	Etretinate. Many other drugs can cause abnormalities, especially if administered between the 8th and 15th weeks of gestation, but there is little exact human data so far. A registry of pregnancies exposed to cancer therapy is maintained by the National Cancer Institute at the University of Pittsburgh.
Testes	Impotence and/or infertility	Alkylating agents, goserelin, leuprolide
	Gynecomastia	Busulfan, estramustine, flutamide
Thyroid	Hypothroidism	Aldesleukin, aminoglutethimide

BIBLIOGRAPHY

Armitage JO, Antman KH, eds, High Dose Cancer Therapy: Pharmacology, Hematopoietins, Stem Cells. Baltimore: Williams & Wilkins, 1992.

Beahrs OH, Henson DE, Hutter RVP, Kennedy BJ, eds, for American Joint Committee on Cancer, Manual for Staging of Cancer, 4th ed. Philadelphia: JB Lippincott, 1992.

Bonadonna G, Robustelli della Cuna G, Handbook of Medical Oncology. Milan: Masson, 1988.

Boring CC, Squires TS, Tong T, Montgomery S, Cancer Statistics, 1994. CA 1994;44:7–26.

Broder S, ed, Molecular Foundations of Oncology. Philadelphia: JB Lippincott, 1991.

Calabresi P, Schein PS, eds, Medical Oncology, 2nd ed. New York: McGraw-Hill, 1993.

Chabner, BA, Collins, JB, eds, Cancer Chemotherapy: Principles and Practice, 2nd ed. Philadelphia: JB Lippincott, 1990.

DeVita VT Jr, Hellman S, Rosenberg SA, eds, Cancer: Principles and Practice of Oncology, 4th ed. Philadelphia: JB Lippincott, 1993.

Dorr RT, Von Hoff DD, Cancer Chemotherapy Handbook, 2nd ed. Norwalk,CT: Appleton & Lange, 1994.

Fischer DS, Knobf MT, Durivage HJ, The Cancer Chemotherapy Handbook, 4th ed. St. Louis: Mosby, 1993.

Fischer DS, Marsh JC, eds, Cancer Therapy. Boston: GK Hall, 1982.

Hoffman R, Benz EJ Jr, Shattil SJ, Furie B, Cohen HJ, eds, Hematology: Basic Principles and Practice. New York: Churchill Livingstone, 1991 (note: 2nd ed, 1994).

Holland JF, Frei E III, Bast RC Jr, Kufe DW, Morton DL, Weichselbaum RR, eds, Cancer Medicine, 3rd ed. Philadelphia: Lea & Febiger, 1993.

Holleb A, Fink DJ, Murphy GP, eds, Textbook of Clinical Oncology. Atlanta: American Cancer Society, 1991.

Hossfeld DK, Sherman CD, Love RR, Bosch FX, eds, UICC Manual of Clinical Oncology, 6th ed. Berlin: Springer-Verlag, 1995.

Lee GR, Bithell TC, Foerster J, Athens JW, Lukens JN, eds, Wintrobe's Clinical Hematology, 9th ed. Philadelphia: Lea & Febiger, 1993.

Miller BA, Ries LAG, Hankey BF, Kosary CL, Harras A, Devasa SS, et al, eds, SEER Cancer Statistics Review 1973–1990. Bethesda: National Cancer Institute, 1993.

Moosa AR, Schimpff SC, Robson MC, eds, Comprehensive Textbook of Oncology, 2nd ed. Baltimore: Williams & Wilkins, 1991.

Nathan DG, Oski FA, eds, Hematology of Infancy and Childhood, 4th ed. Philadelphia: Saunders, 1992.

Niederhuber JE, ed, Current Therapy in Oncology. St. Louis: Mosby, 1993.

Pizzo PA, Poplack DG, eds, Principles and Practice of Pediatric Oncology, 2nd ed. Philadelphia: JB Lippincott, 1993.

Rubin P, ed, Clinical Oncology: A Multidisciplinary Approach for Physicians and Students. Philadelphia: JB Lippincott, 1993.

Stomper PC, Cancer Imaging Manual. Philadelphia: JB Lippincott, 1993.

Tannock IF, Hill RP, eds, The Basic Science of Oncology, 2nd ed. New York: McGraw Hill, 1992.

Wiernik PH, Canellos GP, Kyle RA, Schiffer CA, eds, Neoplastic Diseases of the Blood, 2nd ed. New York: Churchill Livingstone, 1991.

Wingo PA, Tong T, Bolden S, Cancer Statistics, 1995. CA 1995;45:8–30.